Common Sense Healing

James A. May

blue ocean press

tokyo – florida

Published by:
blue ocean press, an imprint of Aoishima Research Institute (ARI)

Main Office (US): P.O. Box 510818, Punta Gorda 33951
Rep. Office: #807-36 Lions Plaza Ebisu , 3-25-3 Higashi, Shibuya-ku, Tokyo, Japan 150-0011

Email: mail@aoishima-research.org

URL: http://www.blueoceanpublications.com
        http://www.aoishima-research.org

ISBN: 978-4-902837-61-2

Acknowledgments

My journey of self discovery has been influenced by too many people to mention them all. However I would not do justice to this book if I did not mention a few of them here. First and foremost I would like to thank my teacher for over 30 years Mr. Prem Rawat Also known as Maharaji who revealed to me the gift of knowledge of my true self. His love and inspiration throughout the years has been a source of strength for me and whose debt I could never repay!

I must also thank Valerie Jean Herth whose love and kindness has kept me alive in one of the darkest periods of my life, and whose love infused me with the will to continue to live! Were it not for her love and kindness I would not have been able to accomplish the healing or the understanding of the recovery process that I present to you here today.

Last, but certainly not least, to my good friend Ken Higgins who has been my rock in time of self-doubt and whose encouragement was of paramount importance to the completion of this book.

To the Brotherhood of Abraham and Lazaris who assisted me in coming to understand the Law of Attraction and Self-Love.

I love them all and I have been blessed to have known them in this life!

James Arthur May
New York, August 2009

Table of Contents

Introduction

In this book I would like to introduce you to a different approach to viewing your body. First and foremost I would like to assist you in coming to the understanding that your body is your best friend! It is also my contention that you have three bodies, a mental body, an emotional body, and a physical body. They are all superimposed on one another. The mental body represents the conscious mind and is a masculine energy. The emotional body represents the subconscious mind and is a feminine energy. And the physical body has the other two superimposed upon it and is a factor that moves through time and space. All three of these bodies have consciousness and communicate with one another. If the communication between these three bodies is harmonious, a person maintains a physical body that is in a state of good health. If there is disharmony between one of these three bodies or all of them, then sickness will manifest.

There is most definitely interplay between these three bodies. They are all of equal value. Many people may be inclined to assign a greater value to the physical body, but they do this to the detriment of the other two bodies. Just as people practice physical hygiene, it would behoove them to practice mental and emotional hygiene as well! Just as viruses may have toxic effect on the physical body, so can toxic thoughts and toxic emotions. If you are sick ask yourself, when is the last time you took time out to evaluate the state of your thoughts and emotions? If you are sick and you are not recovering, there is a good chance some toxic thoughts and emotions have contributed to your being ill. Bringing harmony to the mental and emotional bodies will help the physical body come into balance to resonate with good health and well being.

Chapter 1 – Sickness the Teacher

I was diagnosed with the virus of hepatitis, a disease of the liver. This is a killer virus in its advanced state and has been responsible for the deaths of many people. At the time I was stationed at Fort Dix and was in Walson Army Hospital. The doctors there were on the cutting edge of medicine, and I had access to the most modern treatment facilities and the best treatment that was available at that time in the United States. Although I did not know it at the time, the hepatitis virus had a consciousness of its own and did not want to die. It was determined to live in my body! The treatment I was under was intended to kill this virus but because the virus had a conscious awareness of itself, it mutated to defend itself from the incoming chemicals that were intended to kill it. This virus not only had consciousness, it also had a will to live! The question was this: Was the virus' will to live greater than mine?

I was given a medical discharge from the Army for Chronic Persistent Hepatitis of the Liver. The virus had won the first battle but the war was not over yet! My diagnosis from the Army Doctors was not a promising one and it made me very depressed. They said they had tried everything on me and nothing worked. They said that the possibility of my recovery was not looking very good and at that time I believed them. That was a very big mistake! Then it dawned on me that I was on a life journey. What was life trying to teach me through this disease? And if life was trying to teach me a lesson through this disease, once I learned that lesson could I be healed from the disease? This perspective was a new outlook and approach to my healing process. Could sickness really be a teacher? Could sickness be a tool that life uses to teach you how to live in better harmony with your body?

I wrestled with this question for a very long time. A lot was riding on this question— not just my health and well-being, but my life as well! The doctors had tried their best to help me, but had been unsuccessful. I was sent me home with a prognosis that left me very little hope. They told me, "There is nothing we can do for you. Your situation is hopeless." However there was one factor in this equation that they did not consider: I was not ready to die! At that moment that I decided I was going to be a student. I was going to be a student of my body and the disease that was afflicting it.

I was aware of the fact that the body is a self-healing mechanism, yet somehow this self-healing mechanism could not overcome the affliction of this liver disease. There had to be a reason for that, and I was determined to find out just exactly what the reason was, in order to do that I needed to have a way to initiate a dialogue with my body. I did not have a clue as to how I was going to do that. I thought about this until I thought that my brain was going to explode. Yet I still could not find the answer. The more I thought about it the more frustrated I became, the more frustrated I became, the more my liver began to hurt me. This began to make me very angry and the angrier I became, the sicker I got! All I wanted was for my body to do its job, to do what it was supposed to do and heal itself. But it did not.

As I grew sicker, I no longer went into anger. I bypassed anger and went directly into rage. As this unfolded I watch my body go into jaundice making my complexion turn yellow. I could no longer do the simplest of things. Walking up three flights of stairs or walking anywhere for that matter was very difficult for me. The difficulty of doing the simple things just increased my rage! Could my rage and my disease somehow be intertwined? If this were indeed the case, could my coming to terms with my rage expedite my healing process and assist me in overcoming my disease? I needed answers but where was I supposed to look to find these answers? It seemed like the more I tried to find these answers using my brain, the more I would run up against a brick wall. It was a very frustrating situation, to the point where my jaundice increased, and I was as yellow as a lemon. I began contemplating suicide.

I had a large print Bible sitting on top of the kitchen table. I opened it and my eyes were drawn to the section that said, "Seek and you shall find. Knock and it will be open unto you!" No matter what choices I made, in my heart I knew that suicide was just not the answer. So I prayed and waited for my answer to come. One lesson that life has taught me is that meditation is very good for coping with anger issues. One night while I was sitting in meditation, the light turned on. Prayer is when you talk to that ultimate power, and meditation is where you listen and that power answers you! I was finally connecting the dots; prayer and meditation are heads and tails of the same coin. This understanding would serve me well in the near future.

It had been a few years since my medical discharge from the Army and I was not getting better, however I was not getting any worse. I was living my life in such a way that I had arrested the downward spiral that had been taking place. I had finally accepted the fact that this was a condition that I was probably going to have to live with for the rest of my life, so I decided to make the best of it. This mindset was very beneficial in helping me release my anger and it was this mindset of acceptance that halted my downward spiral! The point I am trying to make here is that while I was in resistance of my disease, that resistance was causing me to become angry.

Consequently I now had two issues to deal with. First was the resistance which the great Carl Jung so eloquently explained with the phrase: "What you resist persists!" And by resisting the situation I could not help but feel angry, and by doing so, I was putting more of this toxic emotion into my body. But more than that my resistance was placing me in the role of a victim, and I was completely disempowering myself! On top of that I still had to deal with what the disease was doing to my body, and how it was making my body feel. I had compounded the problems of my healing process with my resistance and I could not blame anyone else for that. Life was teaching me some very hard lessons through this disease. Anytime I got really angry I would have to stop and rest my body for half an hour. (I mean actually go to bed!) It didn't take much of this for me to finally realize that my body was affected by my emotions, and this is what I mean, when I say the liver is an emotional organ because your emotional states affect your body. Slowly but surely, I was beginning to understand my emotional body. For such a long time the overall condition of my emotional body was anger, because I was resisting the disease in my body. I was beginning to see this quite clearly now. So clearly that one day I was finally able to let it go. *You have this disease,* I thought to myself, *and all the complaining and resisting in the world is not going to change that fact, so accept the fact that you must learn to live with this condition.* When I was finally able to do that, a feeling of peace came over me and I noticed I began to feel a little bit better. I had taken the first step in the right direction towards my healing process by accepting the reality of what is! It was very clear to me now that my emotions affected my body and the state of my health. I recognized that my body was under an assault of toxic emotions and I needed to gain some control over this situation if I was ever going to overcome this disease. What was the source of all of these toxic emotions? Where were they coming from? I had to search for the answers and I discovered the answers were all within me.

The source of all my toxic emotions were coming from the thoughts that I held in my mind stream. In the beginning all of this was running on automatic pilot and I was not aware of the basic principles by which we create through the power of thought and visualization. I was also focusing a great deal of the time on what I did *not* want, which is very harmful to a person. Focusing on anything, even if it is something you *don't* want, will bring that object of your focus right into your actual life experience! Once I became aware of this I began to shift my thoughts from those that were contributing to the promotion of disease and began to focus on what I really wanted – to heal. As men and women we can focus on whatever we want and we do so every day either consciously or unconsciously. The healing mindset is to bring your focus into alignment with what you really want consciously. If I could see myself in a healthy body, I could bring it into manifestation on the physical plane. I know Source-Energy had given me the power to create and what I wanted to manifest was a strong and healthy body. I began to look within myself for the answer. This answer lay in the discovery of my own wisdom, the wisdom that resides in all men and women. When people place themselves in harmony with the divine within them, all healing is possible. This may seem obvious to you, but it was not obvious to me at that time.

I was very good at repressing any emotion that I did not want to feel. I had learned to do this at a very early age because of the child abuse I had suffered. I gave the outward appearance of having my act together, so to speak. But inside I had the emotional maturity of an adolescent! Constant repression of any negative emotions stopped me from developing any kind of real emotional maturity at all. I knew deep down inside of me if I were going to overcome this illness, this repression had to stop. I had to look at myself without repressing anything, to let everything come to the surface, so I could see what was really bothering me. As I did this I was hit with an avalanche of emotion. I was abused as a child and the ramifications of that abuse had continued to that very day. By repressing those emotions the child within me never grew up but he felt safe. But the cost to my body was too high a price to pay for that feeling of safety that the child within me had to have! I could run from myself no longer. I had to fix myself. This was the type of work that no doctor could do for me and I knew it. I had to do this all by myself.

I had come to the understanding that my beliefs are of primary importance in my healing process. I had a very deep-seated belief that I was not worthy and also had very low self esteem. This was totally blocking my healing process and I knew it! So if I were going to heal my body, I needed to start with my mind. I asked myself why. Why do I believe this, why do I believe I am not worthy to be healed? When I opened myself up to this question the answer became quite clear to me, it was because it was beaten into me as a young child. I am not trying to give you a sob story here; I am only trying to make a point. People can't give you what they don't have. My mother did not have the courage to defend me from my stepfather, and my stepfather did not have love in his heart to give me. Neither my mother nor my stepfather were alive at this point in my life, both of them had died a decade earlier. I had been victimized by the actions of my stepfather and the lack of action by my mother. I was determined that I was not going to be a victim any longer! I had suffered enough. I knew that there was suffering in my immediate future, but if I was going to suffer this time, it would be for the right reasons. This time it would be growing pain!

I took the time to sit down and take stock of my emotions and my beliefs. The belief of unworthiness stood out like a sore thumb. This was something I really needed to come to terms with. I realized that my being alive was no accident! I was on a journey of self-discovery. So what was the lesson that life was trying to teach me through this disease? *"LOVE YOURSELF"* was the answer I was given! I needed to open my eyes to the truth of who I truly am.

Let's break down the word *human*. *Hu* comes from the Latin root meaning *light*, and adding *man* means *light man* or *light woman*. And the light that I am and the light that you are, makes us one with the Divine. This makes us all worthy. I am not giving you an intellectual understanding here.

I am giving you a core belief that comes from my innermost being. I am a child of divine energy as are you. There is absolutely nothing, including disease that we cannot overcome! We all have the force of that divine power backing us up. It did not happen overnight but gradually my consciousness began to shift and as it did the unworthiness began to melt away. But this was only the beginning. There was still a long road ahead.

I cannot overstate the importance of self-worth in your healing journey. I speak to you from my very own personal experience. Believing in yourself gives you certain expectations about your life. Allow me expand on this: The beliefs that you have will generate certain thoughts. The thoughts that you hold in your mind stream will generate emotions. These emotions will cause you to have certain

17

feelings. These feelings will cause your body to emanate energy, and like-energy attracts like-energy. (This is an extremely important fact.) Consequently if you feel worthy, your body is emanating a positive energy force. This positive energy force is a magnet and will cause powerful healing energy to return to you, which is precisely what your body wants and needs! You are a powerful being that needs to discover the power that you have within you, both mentally and emotionally. Also the power of your will and the clarity of your intent, this is the missing part of the equation that the doctors cannot provide for you. This is your contribution to your own healing process.

By making this contribution to your healing process you step into your power and begin your dance with the Divine that resides within you. The healing that you desire is just the tip of the iceberg. You have so much power that you can take yourself into good health and well being if you so desire. Most people are not aware of the fact that they are a great contributing factor to their own diseases. The key word here is *aware*. If you are unaware that you are not doing something then you cannot change it.

However once you step into conscious awareness you now have a choice. Become aware of your mental body and the thoughts that flow through it. Are they harmonious healing thoughts that bring peace and tranquility? Or is the opposite the case? I know and believe that you are most definitely worthy of the healing that you desire. What I believe though is inconsequential to your healing process. The important factor is what *you* believe! There is a power that is far greater than you and I, and this power has given you life. This power has blessed you with a human body, and has given you the power of free will and also the power to give and receive love. You are most definitely worthy! It is said that The Lord created the heavens and earth in six days and on the seventh day he rested. It took The Lord nine months to create you! *Nine months!* You are most definitely worthy!

Understanding this mentally is one thing, but understanding this on an experiential level is another thing altogether. For you to understand this on an experiential level, you must do the work. Look inside your mental body to see and understand the overall content of your thoughts. Why do you believe what you believe? How do you think and feel about yourself and your body? This is the first step. Most of us have beliefs but some of us do not know or understand why we believe what we believe. Do not be afraid to take a look inside yourself and find the answers to these questions. By doing so you are taking the steps to understand the power of your mental body.

Doing this will give you a greater insight in understanding why you feel the way you do. It also contributes to your understanding your emotional body.

This brings us to the next step: understanding the emotional body. How do you feel about yourself? How do you *really* feel? Not how you *think* you should feel, but how do you *really* feel about yourself? And however you are truly feeling, be okay with feeling that! If you don't know how you really feel, that's perfectly okay because you can find out. Your emotions create the way you feel and these feelings generate energy. You may be asking yourself what's so important about these feelings and the energy that these emotions generate? Again, like-energy attracts like-energy. If the energy that you are emanating is positive and says *yes* to life, you will attract well-being and good health. However, if the opposite is true, you will attract sickness.

It is just common sense! You have a choice in this matter. Use the power of your mind and emotions to assist you in manifesting healing energy and good health, because you have the power to do so. Every single human being on the planet is blessed with this power. Weather they realize it or not, they still have it, and this includes you also! Step into your power and say *yes* to your healing and *yes* to life. You can do it because you are most definitely worthy!

Chapter 2 – Your Best Friend

After my medical discharge I left Fort Dix and returned to New York. It was at that point that I realized how debilitating the sickness of Chronic Hepatitis C really is. This sickness is very deceptive. One of the extreme side effects of hepatitis is that your skin can turn yellow. But unless you manifest that extreme side effect you look perfectly healthy. But no one with an unhealthy liver is really healthy. I found this out rather quickly when I tried to go to work. Physical labor was out of the question. I just couldn't do it! Being a very active person, that sounded like a death sentence to me. This was the cause of great frustration within me. I had no idea of the best way to process my emotions (of which anger was the most predominant). Rather than embracing the anger and making it my own, I repressed it. This was not a very wise way to deal with it. As a matter of fact, it was the worst thing I could have done!

At that time, I did not understand the relationship between my mind, my emotions and my body. I also did not realize that the liver is an emotional organ, and anger is a very toxic emotion for it. I was on a healing journey to recovery and there was still much that the disease of hepatitis had to teach me, about myself *and* my body. That's right. Sickness can be a teacher and it can be a great teacher if you are open to see the lessons that lie within you.

When I was finally able to accept this as a truth in my life an exciting sense of self-discovery was awakened within me. It feels good to be fulfilling the purpose of this life – to have the smile that needs no explanation, the quite smile of the heart enjoying each and every breath being given to me by the mother of all life.

This body is a self-healing mechanism. It will heal itself automatically. This is not something you need to think about, because thinking involves conscious thought. The self-healing power of the body is regulated by the subconscious mind which is beyond the scope of conscious thought.

However, if one can have the subconscious *and* conscious mind working in tandem, it is my belief that any disease can be healed. Please don't misunderstand what I'm trying to say here. Sickness is a part of life.

Human beings get sick, animals get sick, plants and trees contract diseases and die. There are also some predispositions in your family gene pool that make you prone to some sicknesses more than others. There are also seasonal viruses that cause us to become sick. However, I'm sure all of you know someone who is always on the go, always moving, and rarely sick.

Ask them how they're doing and they will tell you they're doing great. Even if they should get sick the recovery time is far less for them than it is for most other people. Why is this? This is because these people have developed a relationship with their best friend, their body! It is said in the Bible that the body is a temple. How are you treating your temple? How are you treating your best friend? Do you even know that your body is your best friend?

Getting back to the interplay between the mental, emotional, and physical bodies, as I stated earlier, I had lots of anger. When I started to see this anger come up, I began to notice the frequency at which it occurred. I experienced this emotion constantly. This was a red flashing light but at the time I did not know it. I had to budget my energy and strength for the smallest task and this was very frustrating! Going to shop at the supermarket seemed to like one of the 12 labors of Hercules, and this also made me angry. I was beginning to see how this was disempowering me because it was the strongest emotion emanating from my emotional body. This emotion of anger was placing me in conflict with myself! I began to spiral into a deep depression, but this was a good thing because I learned from it. What I learned was that depression is my anger turned inward and directed at me! I knew that I needed to come to terms with this situation, because the results of my *not* coming to terms with it meant death! If there were ever a candidate for an anger management course, I would be on the top-ten list.

At this point in my life I was in my early 30s – the

prime of life for most people. That was not the case with me. I felt that my life was over at 30, and I could feel myself losing my desire to live. Life was becoming too hard.

Rather than live this way, I knew the one thing I had total control over was the termination of my own life. There was just one problem: Although life was extremely difficult, I was just not ready to die. I began to realize that I needed to empower myself!

When I had left Walson Army Hospital at Fort Dix, my prognosis was not a very good one. I had been told there was nothing that they could do for me. These were highly trained doctors telling me that there was no hope for me and I was foolish enough to believe them. (After all, they were *doctors!)* But through my daily introspection and meditation sessions, I became acutely aware of the fact that as long as there is life there is hope, no matter what the doctors tell you! God gives miracles each and every day to his children, and I was going to receive one of these miracles.

In the army and through the practice of martial arts I realized the power of focusing the mind. Although I never intentionally focused my mind on healing my body, I used the power of focus primarily in breaking boards or visualizing hitting the center of the bull's-eye. I realized that if I was going to empower myself I needed to focus my mind on the fact that I could be healed! So what if the doctors could not help me? There is a higher power in control of all of this and that power is not controlled by the doctors. Put yourself in harmony with universal law, and you can be the recipient of this power. I believed this then and I believe this now. I am one of many who are living testament to that fact.

Belief is of utmost importance in the healing process of any major disease. It is my firm belief that anytime a major disease manifests in your life, you have come to a crossroad. Some important factor for your development and evolutionary growth must be dealt with. Believe it or not, my disease was a teacher to me and I learned lessons through my disease that I would never have learned otherwise. It is my firm belief that once a person has learned the lessons that a sickness is trying to teach, then that sickness no longer serves a purpose being in the body! When whatever factors that are blocking a person's development and evolutionary growth have been overcome, the body can then restore itself back into harmony and good health.

If you are anything like me, your personal beliefs will be of paramount importance to you in accomplishing this. I realized very early in my journey that some of my beliefs were healthy and promoted healing. However, some of my beliefs were extremely toxic and could promote sickness and even death. A brutally honest self evaluation was the foundation on which I would create the new me but my evaluation, although brutally honest, was also kind, fair and loving. I believe to the core of my very being that my disease manifested as my teacher to teach me some vitally important lessons. This belief gave me power, strength and the courage to say yes to life. A person can either choose life, or choose death, and your beliefs are an indicator of your choice.

As a result of my meditations, I could see I was operating in what I call *victim mode*. There is one thing of which I am 100% sure. When I operate in *victim mode* I completely and totally disempowered myself. A victim fails to realize his or her own power. That also includes the potential to heal.

When a person is in *victim mode*, he or she attracts toxic thoughts and emotions, most of which are totally disempowering. What I am talking about here is the capacity to do your own mental, emotional, and physical hygiene. Be aware of your mind, and the thoughts that you mind produces. As you do this you move into the realm of mental hygiene. How do your thoughts make you feel? Good-feeling thoughts promote healing. With bad-feeling thoughts the opposite is true. Thoughts and feelings are like heads and tails of the same coin; they go together. Your thoughts create your feelings and your feelings motivate you to act. If I think that someone has done me an injustice, those thoughts can bring me to anger, and that anger may cause me to take action. Most actions that are taken under the influence of anger are not beneficial to us or other people. So the thoughts and feelings that we have about ourselves and others do influence our actions. My question to you is this: How do you think and feel about yourself? How do you think and feel about your body? Because how you feel about your body and how you think about it will be a good indicator of how you are treating your best friend.

I cannot overstate the importance of your feelings in relation to your healing process. If you have a strong feeling of self-worth, then you probably feel that you deserve to be healed. However, if the opposite is the case, you probably have a strong feeling that you do not deserve to be healed. The most important factor in your healing process is your mind! And when I say your mind, I mean the entire mind, both conscious and subconscious.

You may be thinking to yourself, I have a hard enough time with just my thoughts! Now this guy is telling me I have to manage my mind! That is *not* what I am saying. You do the best you can to be on top of your thinking process. In that step it's all about your conscious mind and you consciously observing your thoughts. Then there are some techniques that will assist you in influencing the content of your subconscious mind. The subconscious mind is important because the subconscious mind runs and maintains the body.

There was an experiment that was done with hypnotherapy. The patient was hypnotized and under the influence of hypnosis and the therapist said to the patient, "I'm going to touch your hand with the tip of a lit cigarette." In reality, what the therapist had done was to touch the patient's hand with the tip of a pencil eraser. As this was done a blister immediately appeared on the patient's hand! If the patient had been conscious and not under hypnosis, this could not have happened, because the person would have seen that they were merely being touched with a pencil eraser. But because the person was under hypnosis, the therapist had access to the subconscious mind of that person.

The subconscious mind believed that the body was being touched with a lit cigarette and responded accordingly, even though it was only a pencil eraser. This is the power of the subconscious mind! We shall tap into this power together. It is not an impossible task. Then you may direct and influence your subconscious in the way you see fit. Then you will become your own *Holistic Doctor* and you and your medical doctor can work in tandem. You will be sitting in the driver's seat and the doctor will be riding shotgun next to you on the passenger side.

To be in the driver's seat is to take control of your life and instruct the doctor regarding your wishes! Many people give their power away to their doctors. They visit the doctor with the attitude of "*The doctor will fix me*". And they refuse to take any responsibility for their healing process.

They will do almost anything the doctor says without question! My question to you is: Who knows your body better than you do? What I am talking about is a mindset that will bring you into your own personal power (Whether you have tapped into it yet or not, you *do* have it!).

I began to look within to discover my true power. Many times in my life I have lost sight of the inner journey that accompanies me in this dance through time and space. When that happens I just return my focus to that truth that vibrates within me. It is the knowledge of all knowledge, to know the truth within you. When you hear that truth you will know because your heart knows the truth. That is because that truth also resonates within you.

Experiencing that truth will help you heal your heart, as it did mine. I have a love in my heart for the truth. There is power in that truth and there is power in my love for it! The power of love for the knowledge I have received is beyond words. I know that I have no greater gift than the gift of this life!

This appreciation of my life gives me a sense of gratitude. I am watching my life unfold like a rose in the morning sun. I am surrounded by this vibrating energy pulsating throughout everything, including me! I am conscious of this fact because I have also been given the gift of consciousness! The blessings bestowed upon each and every one of us are there if we but open our eyes to them. If you can do this, you will open an express lane to healing and happiness in your life. Source Energy also gives us the power to give and receive love. Then we also have been given this faithful companion – a human body. What a magnificent apparatus to experience life with on this earth! This body is my true best friend. Even though I have abused it, it has always stuck by me and will stick by me to the end. Now *that's* a friend!

The day came when I lay in my bed contemplating the coming morning. I was going to the hospital for liver biopsies. I was going to use all the tools I had available to use and modern medicine was also one of them. I will spare you the details of that following morning. It's enough to say it will never be on my list of favorite things to do! I came home after the procedure and it was coming home to an empty house that slapped me in the face. This one hurt! I was alone. I wanted a companion in my life and all I had was myself and my sickness! I stayed away from people. This again forced me to go within to discover my own power: the life force energy I take in through the power of my breath moment by moment. Oh, what a joy it is! I am alive because of it. Oh what a blessing! What a gift! This experience gave me the will to live and the power to go on. After about 18 months I was no longer contagious so now I could be around people once again, but I had lost the desire. I was on disability so my income was very limited and I had done a pretty good job of isolating myself, so I had few friends. I was lonely sometimes but I was never alone. The knowledge of that truth that vibrates within gives me inner strength. I am one with that Ultimate Power and that Power is one with me. There is nothing together we cannot do! I must have my miracle; I must manifest my healing. I owe it to my best friend!

The results from the liver biopsies were not promising and at this point I had decided no more hospitals, no more tests and no more doctors. I was going down my own path and was going to take the road less traveled!

From now on, no one's advice was going to be of greater value to me in my own life than the advice I got from my own heart! I decided I was going to heal myself! I was going to watch my miracle unfold, as it did!

I decided to go back to the basic theme that you are what you eat. I began eating brown rice and veggies, fish and sometimes a little chicken. I really felt good from eating the brown rice, salads and veggies. I actually liked it. My body is so much more intelligent than I am! It helps me by making me crave what is good for me. When I listen to my body and feed it what it is asking for, it thanks me. It is grateful to me as I am grateful to it, my best friend! I also started taking an interest in hands-on healing. I knew that a woman was going to come into my life to reveal something to me that would be very important. I was hoping for a romantic interest but I just wasn't feeling that.

When I met her I would know. (Something inside me already knew this!) It was time to shop for a few things so I went to the Mall. I needed to pick up some socks and some briefs. While I was looking through some socks I felt someone's gaze upon me. As I looked up I saw a woman looking at me. She had a very serene look about her and a light in her eyes that was very soothing and comforting. It was her and I knew it! All of a sudden I had butterflies in my stomach. I felt like I was back in high school. Something was telling me to just run away! But I knew I could not let my insecurities get the better of me here; at least I had to try to talk to her! But what was I going to say? I had no idea! My palms became moist, and all of a sudden my mouth was as dry as sandpaper. As I walked toward her I thought she must hear my heart pounding through my chest! All I could muster was, "Hello." As if she saw the great effort that it took for me, she smiled and said, "Hello." I said, "I think we are supposed to talk." "I believe you are right," she answered. I asked her, "May I buy you a cup of coffee?" "No," she said, "but you may buy me a cup of black jasmine tea." "That's my favorite tea also," I told her. I felt comfortable and safe with this raven- haired beauty. "Do you know what we are to talk about," she asked?"I have opened my mind to the possibility of accessing my healing energy," I started to say to her, but before I could finish the

32

sentence, she said "It's you! I had a different picture of you in my mind but your energy tells me that you are the one!" This woman told me of things to come and things I had the potential to accomplish. As we spoke I saw something in her eyes looking back at me that I saw in myself. There was a mutual recognition between travelers on the same path!

As we sat down to talk for a moment she told me, "Jimmy, you have the gift. And you can also help people heal, but first you must heal yourself!" She saw the pain in my heart. "You must come to terms with your pain so you may heal," she said. The fact that she saw my heart and spoke to me so gently, with so much kindness brought a tear to my eye. Women can be so beautiful sometimes! This type of treatment was new to me and I could feel its healing effect. We spoke for about 20 minutes, and then the person she was waiting for showed up and she was gone. I have never seen her again! Yet the impact of that brief encounter remains with me to this day. Her beauty was truly profound, I am not talking about her looks although she was very pleasing to look at, and she had this peaceful air about her. What I am talking about is her energy! Her demeanor was soft-spoken and quiet, yet she had a powerful presence of energy surrounding her. Her words gave insight to the new path that was unfolding for me. This was an inner journey: Heal the mind and the body will follow!

"*Know Thyself*," said the great Socrates. Is there

knowledge of the self? I ask myself could there be something within me that needs to be known and, if so, where would that something be? I have discovered for myself that the consciousness in my body rides on the wind of the breath! This has been my experience. Through the power of a most beautiful and simple placement of my attention on the breath, and I can plug into my source. I can see that I have the power to manifest all the things I need. This body is of absolute importance to me maintaining my existence on this earth! I must place myself in harmony with universal law and by doing so the higher vibration energy frequencies become available to my body. I could see that I was evolving in consciousness; higher energy was now entering into me through my meditations. I was expanding my consciousness and my body needed to follow suit! That night as I sat alone I decided to turn off the TV. I sat in silence for a moment then I placed my left hand on my navel and my right on my heart. A pleasing flow of warm energy began to flow through my body and I could channel it to my hands. "Oh, my God," I thought to myself, the raven haired beauty was right! This is so cool I thought to myself! I sat there for about 20 minutes sending this energy to my body. When I finished I fell out for about two hours and I slept like a rock. After the rest I got up and saw my reflection in the mirror, I looked visibly better even to my own eyes and I am a tough critic.

That night I had a long and needed good night's sleep. I jumped out of bed the next morning without noticing how much extra energy I had. I made myself my morning tea and sat down at the kitchen table. I was realizing that the wake up fog was lifting much quicker than usual, and I was really enjoying the cup of black jasmine tea. Its taste and aroma were pleasing to me and not being in that wake up fog allowed me to be conscious and appreciate the simple pleasure of a morning cup of tea! I was having some inner dialogue with myself about the previous night events. I wonder if it was just wishful thinking on my part, after all I am just like everyone else; does everyone have the capacity to tap into this energy to heal? At that point I was not sure but I was going to find out.

I took time to find a quite place to mediate. I am sharing with you something that is very special to me in my life. To have knowledge of the power that resides within the Breath brings a feeling of gratitude to my heart. I love gratitude because gratitude helps my body heal. Gratitude is to my sprit what vitamin-C is to the body! I like to take it in large dosages! My meditation brought me to a quite place, my thoughts were now quietly in the background and I could hear the voice and guidance of my inner self! Again just as the night before I placed my left hand over my navel and my right hand over my heart, again the warm pleasing energy began to flow me. Just like the night before I sent this energy into my body for about 20 minutes.

Again I fell asleep soundly for 2 hours. Upon awakening, I knew I had tap into something very powerful. I was going to see if I could use it as a tool in my dance with my disease.

I decided I was going to program myself with a new habit through the power of my will! I was going to give myself one 20 minutes session in the morning and one 20 minute session in the evening also. Every day for one month I would keep a journal so I could see my own thoughts and feelings on my movement through this 30 day process. This was a cleansing process; however it is a two-fold process, a cleansing of mind and also body. To tell you that this process was blissful would be false, it was sometimes and sometimes it can be downright painful. Understand what I mean when I say painful. What could be painful about sending energy into your body and keeping a journal for 30 days? Sometimes the energy blockages are not just mental they can be emotional as well. When a repressed emotional blockage something that you have consciously been choosing not to deal with, manifests in your mind stream of thought; your emotional body is telling you it's time to let it go! Your mind, your higher mind will not allow you to repress it any longer because it is now an obstacle to your evolutionary growth process! It has been my experience that these obstacles usually come in clusters. This is where you are pushed beyond your comfort zone and one has the sensation of things falling apart! However when you deal with these obstacles you expand in consciousness and so does the threshold of your comfort zone! By doing this you step into a higher level of self awareness, and also start stepping into your true power!

Being unemployed gave me a lot of free time and I decided to use this time wisely. I was hungry for knowledge, self-knowledge, healing knowledge and the knowledge of the universal laws of the earth plane. By this time I now understood at this point in my healing journey the relationship between the conscious and subconscious mind. I knew at that point that my conscious and subconscious mind both think in pictures and I could influence them both by the pictures I visualized; I was not powerless anymore! Although I was aware of this before, it was just information at the time. I needed to know how this information could be valuable to me on my healing journey.

I was having a lot of dreams. A few of these dreams I just could not forget! The emotions I felt around these dreams and the fact that I could not forget them told me that the messages that they contain were very important and of great value to me. I had a sense that my subconscious mind was communicating to me through the dream state! I decided I ought to learn how to interpret my dreams. That's exactly what I did. I have received guidance, warnings and information about my body all through the dream state. I like everyone else had been dreaming my entire life. I've never looked at my dreams as a tool to help me in my healing process until then.

Many times I would dream about certain events that happened in my past. Usually they were situations in which I had been traumatized as a young boy! For a long time I resisted having these dreams. When I would wake up the following morning after these dreams, many times I would be drenched in sweat and my heart would be pumping like crazy! I thought I was having bad dreams, nightmares. However this was not the case! My subconscious mind was desperately trying to assist me in my healing process through these dreams. My subconscious mind was telling me that I needed to work on these traumatizing situations that had traumatized me when I was a young boy. I had to look at the content of this trauma that was in my dreams in order to release and let go of it! It is very important for me to understand this key point! I am not saying that a person has to relived the trauma of their past, just look at it with the intention of letting it go!

I cannot overstate the importance of your dreams. Let me illustrate the point I'm trying to make with an example. I was in upstate New York on a retreat. I went to the hotel dining room for a buffet breakfast. I made myself a plate of food and began to search for place to sit. I saw a table with one place available. I asked the people at the table, was that seat available and they said yes. By the conversation I could see that the people at the table all knew each other and we're friends. One man was talking about a dream he had the night before. He was telling his friends that he was very perverted because of this dream he had. In the dream he was wearing a trench coat and walks up to his wife and flashed her; he was naked underneath the trench coat! He was boasting about how sick he had behaved in his dream. Then he said no wonder she wants to divorce me! At this point I said to him, that is a very beautiful dream Sir! He looked at me with great anger and said what on earth are you talking about? Show me how this is a good dream! All his friends were now focused on me also. They were just waiting for to explain that statement and if they didn't like the explanation I knew that I was going to be verbally attacked. Sir I said you are in the process of getting a divorce is that correct? Yes he replied. You really don't want this divorce do you?

No he answered. Your higher self is talking to through this dream I told him. This is what your dream is trying to tell you. The opening up of your trench coat is symbolic and what is good about it is that it is telling you that you need to reveal yourself to your wife in total emotional nakedness–not physical nakedness! Instead of playing this happy-go-lucky role and pretending that absolutely nothing is bothering you. You must reveal your naked emotion to your wife; allow her to witness the pain you feel in losing her and your sons. Allow her to know that you are willing to do whatever is in your power to save your family. Stop pretending that nothing is bothering you. If you want to keep you family you must reveal yourself to your wife in complete emotional nakedness! As I said this I watched the anger completely drain out of him. He had an overwhelmed look on his face. I sat quietly for a moment to give him a minute to recover from what I had said.

He was becoming a little emotional and I could see was trying to fight back some tears. I don't want my sons to call another man dad he said! It would kill me to lose my wife and my boys! You must be brave and share this with your wife she will love you for it! It will make the bond between the two of you much stronger I said. You are still in time to save your marriage I told him. She is a good woman your wife and you know that. She is worth all the effort you must make to try to keep her. Your dam right she is he replied! I was finished with my breakfast and it was time to start my day. I excused myself from the table and stood up. As I did so, so did the man I was talking to and extended his hand to me to shake hands. As I shook his hand he gave me a hug so tight it hurt. Thank you I don't know where you came from but I am sure glad I met you he said! This is how your subconscious mind can communicate to you through the dream state!

Because of the condition of my liver I was very susceptible to colds and viruses. I caught a bad virus that put on my back for two weeks. This made me very depressed and the toxic thoughts in my mind stream were telling me that it was no use, my situation was hopeless. I decided that I needed to go into the meditation to find some answers, but first, I prayed. My life journey has taught me that prayer is when you talk to Source Energy and meditation is where Source Energy answers you! I asked myself what I am doing wrong. I have been wrestling with this disease for a while now yet I am still unable to heal. What is the lesson that life is trying to teach me through the sickness, I asked myself? Then I sat down, closed my eyes and meditated. I meditated for about an hour and a half and when I was done I felt much better. I had gotten my answer. The answer was, when you learn the lesson that this sickness is trying to teach you, you shall be healed. However I needed to discover that answer for myself! It was at point that I enrolled in the school of life, so to speak. I was majoring in understanding my disease I had to, my life depended on it! Let me interject a very important point here, maybe your personal issue is not with anger like mine was, perhaps your issue is with grief, or guilt, maybe it is with fear or anxiety! No matter what the emotions of your personal issue are this approach to your healing can be of great benefit to you if you only give it a chance. Whatever your personal issue is please do not dismiss this information because your issue is not with anger, because if you do so you are not seeing the big picture! The big picture is that you are just like the rest of us human beings and as human beings we are all affected by our thoughts and emotions. When you begin to make an effort to use the power of your will to consciously examine the content of your thoughts and emotions, then you begin to change the energy frequency of your body's resonation! As a result you begin to emanate an energy frequency from both the mental and emotional plane that is putting out a difference signal to "Source Energy". This new signal is now telling the universe that you are ready to look at the factors that are blocking your healing process and evolutionary growth! You see we communicate verbally however we also communicate energetically as well, and this energetic communication is much more powerful than the verbal and is picked up by Source-Energy and acted upon! Using the power of your will and the clarity of your intention you are now sending a clear signal out into the universe of what you want, and the universe will now respond in kind. As a result of going through this process there will be a gradual transition from seeing your body as a sickness machine, to now seeing your body as having the potential to heal. As it gradually begins to heal then you can make the transition to seeing it as your best friend. You see you can't love a sickness machine-but you can love your best friend! This

42

may seem totally unimportant to you; however when an actual shift in consciousness takes place in your mind stream; that shift brings in a new aspect of now viewing your body as your friend. This shift in your mindset will advance your healing progress exponentially.

Chapter 3 – Consciousness Communicates
With Consciousness

I was unable to work due to my liver cancer therefore I was spending a lot of time at home alone. My doctor thought it would be a good idea to get some hobbies. I went with cooking, tropical fish and music, and I really like cooking! I met my girlfriend who was a tropical fish lover, and an excellent teacher. She has taught how to take care of the tropical fish. Together we set up two fish tanks, a 55 gallon and a 30 gallon tank. The tanks were beautiful with colorful and vibrant fish, each with their own personality vibrating with life force energy just like you and me. We would talk to each other just not verbally! You see I have consciousness and so do the fish and consciousness communicates with consciousness! It's just a matter of common sense because if your line of communication is open, an exchange of communication can take place! What about the line of communication with my body? Could I communicate energetically with my body just like I was learning to do with these fish? I wondered what my body would say to me. I knew I was going to redefine my relationship with my body. The person I was who was unaware of how my actions affected my body had to die, so the new me could be resurrected! I spent the major part of the morning cleaning the fish tanks. It was work to clean the tanks but so worth it because they are magical panoramic gifts of Mother Nature's beauty in my living room, how sweet it is!

I just finished making dinner and went to sit down in the living room. I was looking for the remote to turn on the TV, as I looked over to my right I could see the fish in the tank trying to swim towards me, to get my attention. I just finished making lasagna for dinner, and I was quite comfortable on the couch and didn't exactly want to get up, so I didn't! That is when I learned the lesson that consciousness communicates with consciousness. As I looked at the fishes in the tank, they all bunched up in the corner that was nearest me.

The fish began to swim in a little formation, all five of them. I got their message loud and clear. I thought they were all very hungry! It was not yet their dinner time. But in my gut I strongly felt they were hungry. So I decided to test the accuracy of my gut felt intuition. I walked over to the fish tank. As I was getting up from the couch, I noticed the fish getting noticeably more excited. As I got closer to the tank, they began to swim from the bottom of the tank to the top. When I reached the tank, I lifted up the hood. The fishes were already opening and closing their mouths in anticipation of the food I was about to send into the tank. Having confirmed the feeling in my gut that my fishes were hungry, I fed them! Shortly after I fed the fishes my girlfriend returned home from work. The feeding activity of the fishes in the fish tank caught her attention. It was then that she said to me, I'm really glad you fed the fishes Jimmy. I was running late for work this morning. I had to run out of the house without feeding them! This brought a smile to my face. She asked me what was so funny, and I told her about the rap session I just had with the angel fishes. She smiled and said it's about time. I told you they talk to you! You just had to learn how to listen!

The point I am trying to make here is that I am a living conscience being in a human body, just as the fishes are living conscience beings in the body of fish. Consciousness communicates with consciousness. People have consciousness, dogs have consciousness. Cats have consciousness, fish have consciousness. Sickness also has consciousness!

You just needed to learn how to listen was what Mallory had said to me, that phrase stuck with me! As we sat down to dinner, Mallory told me about her day. As I sat across from her I wondered what I had done to deserve such a beautiful woman in my life. Hey Mal I said, after dinner, can we talk? Sure she answered. After dinner, we cleared the dinner table together, and then sat down to talk. So what's up, she asked me? I said, when I spoke to you about my rap session with the fishes, you told me I just needed to learn how to listen! Please explain that for me. What exactly did you mean? Jimmy she said the fish are intelligent and are smarter than you think. They didn't have breakfast this morning, so they were hungry. You had no way of knowing that. The fish knew what they needed to do. All five of them were hungry.

They communicated with one another and decided that they were going to collaborate together. And that's exactly what they did! First they all swam in formation coming towards you, next collectively all five of them began to send you their energy at the same time. And when you finally got up from the couch and began to walk towards the tank, they all began to swim from the bottom to the top of the tank, opening and closing their mouths in a feeding frenzy. At this point, even you knew that they were hungry! Mother Nature has given us all a way to communicate and express ourselves. You just need to tune in and learn how to listen. You're in the process of learning that right now.

I wanted to better understand my body consciousness to expedite my healing process. New possibilities were opening up for me to understand and communicate with other living things without the use of language! I began to develop the capacity to listen. Then to answer back; the dialog between my body and I was a catalyst in understanding this process. I began to ask myself questions like how do I communicate with my body? Is there any communication at all happening or am I so wrap up in my life that I do not have time to listen to my body? I was not happy with all the answers I got but asking the questions put me one step closer to my healing, and also gave me a clear picture of where I was standing in relation to my here and now!

That clarity gave me the power of wisdom and choice. You don't have to accept whatever the mind throws at you base on a fear based belief system! I say again, you don't have to accept whatever your mind throws at you based on a fear based belief system!

There was a time as children when we were afraid of the dark. Today we have all outgrown that belief system and have new ones. The question is; is your belief system working for you? You see I began to change my consciousness by changing my beliefs. And I started with the little things first like believing I could communicate with my fish or my cats, dogs and other animals without the use of language. I was in constant communication with my body now and sensitive to its messages. Slowly I began to see an improvement, not a whole lot but it was a step in the right direction! You see what motivates me on my journey is the will to live and to witness the unfolding of the development of my own consciousness! It is one of the many gifts in my life. I see this life as a learning process and sickness is really an opportunity to get back in touch with the basics. The Sprit within us wants to live in good health and not only that it wants to dance! Have you felt your sprit lately? You see consciousness communicates with consciousness and my sprit wanted to know the consciousness that creates all things. That consciousness could instruct me on how to bring my body back into balance and good health. You see I was and am clear on what I want when it comes to my body – Good Health! The biggest factor in healing your body is you, even though your body is a self-healing mechanism it is influenced by the power of your thought! There is just no way out of it; your mind influences your body. Listen to and know the type of incoming thoughts you and your body must contend with each and every day. We want to do this to see if the thoughts we have are toxic. You can picture it as pulling weeds from your garden in preparation to plant fruits or flowers. The key here is just to observe what is going on without any judgment. Whatever thoughts and feelings come up let them and just watch, do not do anything else, just allow the thoughts and feelings to be there. You do not have to step into those feelings if they are painful! Just be aware of what going on within your mind and how those thoughts and those feelings make you feel.

Remember this is a process so go at your own pace. The key here is to be okay with whatever you are feeling and give to yourself the same love you would like to receive from others when you put yourself through this process! If you can keep a light hearted attitude you can have fun with this- yes fun! This is your journey of self discovery and you can make it fun or a great pain, the choice is yours!

At this point I would like to address a few issues about sickness and mental body. There are some sicknesses that affect us and are outside of our control. For example all of us have the capability of catching a cold. Every winter flu season comes, and although none of us want to catch the flu we are all susceptible to these viruses and can catch them and become sick from time to time. This is just a simple fact of life, and comes with the territory if you are alive on the earth plane! There are mistakes we can make such as not putting on the proper amount of clothing in cold weather and we can get sick. However the point I would like to make here is that it is my contention that a person can catch a cold or the flu-but you just don't catch Cancer or Lupus and Hepatitis, even if you have a predisposition because of hereditary factors on your family tree. I believe these major diseases develop over time and that they do not manifest magically over night! I am a firm believer that the thoughts you allow to occupy the consciousness of your mental body are one of the major contributing factors to the development of disease! I speak from my own personal experience. When I began to make a serious attempt to become conscious of the thought processes of my mental body, I began to recognize how these thoughts were making me feel. Some of these thoughts were healthy thoughts and promoted healing, and some were totally toxic and were contributing to the manifestation of disease! However when I became conscious of these thoughts and emotions I now had the power of choice. I chose to perform my mental and emotional hygiene, and took responsibility for my healing. This was an activity that no doctor could perform for me, and no doctor can perform for you! Step into your power because you are not powerless against your disease. Consciousness or better put a lack of consciousness may manifest your illness. However by stepping into your conscious awareness you become the "Holistic Doctor" of your own consciousness, now you are working with two doctors, you're medical doctor who will work with your physical body and you who will work with your consciousness! Now you have both barrels of the healing shotgun working in tandem, and this increases the odd of a healing in your favor.

This is what common sense healing is all about. Step into your common sense consciousness and grow. Manifest the miracle you so desperately want and need. Do not give your power away to the doctor and make it the doctor's responsibility to fix you! Step into your own power and work in tandem with your doctor and watch your miracle unfold! If your doctor is uncooperative then get another doctor, but in most cases you will be surprised to see how cooperative you doctor will be. We are all in earth school and one of the lessons we need to learn is how to correct our body's imbalances to maintain good health. Good health is your birth right and you deserve it. Know it, believe it, and have the faith that Source-Energy will guide you to the understanding that you need to manifest your healing, I am living proof that this can happen!

The emotions that we experience along with our thoughts are also a great contributing factor to the status of our health. In this day and age many women suffer from breast cancer. It is my firm belief that the emotions that are experienced via the emotional body are also a contributing factor in the manifestation of breast cancer, and science has confirmed the mind body relationship! Let say that a woman is in a relationship with a man and he betrays her; he has sex with her best friend. Not only does the woman have to deal with the betrayal of her man, but also of her so called best friend!

Plus the humiliation that comes with this situation of friends and associates who may also know that this has happen to her. There is a good chance that she may be overwhelmed by all the toxic emotions this situation can produce. Needless to say she has also a broken heart. If she does not process these emotions properly, the toxic emotions will build up and she could very well manifest cancer of the breast! Her broken heart is also located in her breast area! I hope you can see the relationship here. I believe that we have not yet found a cure for cancer because there are multiply factors that contribute to its manifestation! It is my belief that the content of our emotional bodies is one those major contributing factors to disease. This just makes good common sense! A man does not get a double pneumonia when he asks his girl friend to marry him and she says yes! But his chances of getting pneumonia if she says no are greater because of what is now going on within his emotional body; stress, sadness, disappointment, and rejection. It is my contention that our emotions play a key role in the maintenance of good health. Science has now confirmed the mind, body connection as well! I hope you can see the common sense of this logic. If you can monitor your thoughts and emotions you can greatly increase your chances of staying healthy, and of recovering from illness if in fact you do get sick. And the wisdom to do this already lies within you; you just need to tap into it by using your common sense!

Our bodies have intelligence, and consciousness. Our bodies understand what to do to keep us healthy. If you doubt that your body has consciousness consider this, when a person is asleep the brain is at rest but if the body is in an uncomfortable position it automatically adjust itself! You are asleep and not even aware that your body is doing this, but your best friend-your body is taking of you even as you sleep. We tend to take these things for granted but stop for just a moment and consider the amount of love that Source-

Energy has placed in your body's natural process just for you! We are all magnificent human beings on a journey of self discovery to discover the Divine within us. Once you realize this and tap into your Divinity there is no sickness that cannot be overcome!

Please understand what I am saying here; we all come into the earth by the process of birth, and exit the earth by the process death. This is true for all living things not just you and I, we all must die. However the quality of life and health that we experience while we are here is entirely up to us! We are creators who have been given free will by Source-Energy and if we have unwittingly created illness we have the power to change that and make health and well being a reality in our life! Understand how great a gift and blessing the consciousness of your mind truly is. Everything you see around you; this book, the chair you are sitting on, the home you are living in all started out as a thought in someone mind first. Use the power of conscious thought to impregnate your mind with the seed of good health. I am talking about taking control of your life through the power of your conscious thought. However this will require a change in how you are currently doing things. But if you know one thing it is that you have the power to change!

Remember that this is a process and it may take you a little time to understand it, but you have the common sense to master it. The choice is entirely up to you.

There is an energy that vibrates your body and gives it life. We call this energy your life force energy. Whether you realize it or not you have the capability to use and manipulate this energy, because it is after all your energy! When this energy flows freely the body maintains a state of health, when it does not sickness occurs. Negative thoughts and emotions have the capability to create blockages to the flow of this energy within the body.

How you think and feel can affect the flow of this energy as well. Consequently how you think and feel is of the utmost importance in maintaining a healthy body. If you place your thoughts and attention on your sickness, you are sending energy to the sickness! I say again, if you place your thoughts and attention on your sickness you are sending energy to the sickness! The point I'm trying to make here is when you get on the telephone and talked to your spouse or friend about your sickness for an hour or so, you are sawing the branch that you are sitting on! You have spent one of hour of your life and one hour of your life force energy in talking about your illness. And you have given your life force energy to your sickness in talking about it. As a result of doing so you have made your disease stronger! If you really want to heal do not do this! Even if you spouse or friend calls you to ask you how you are doing, because he or she may be genuinely be concerned about you. Understand what I am saying here, I am not saying don't talk to your spouse or friend, just be conscious of what you talk to them about! If you are focusing on your sickness and talking about your sickness you are going to attract more sickness! It is of critical importance to your healing process that you understand this! With just a subtle shift in your awareness from sickness to wellness you can make a quantum leap towards good health. Spend that hour talking to your spouse or friend about your wellness. I use the term wellness here for a good reason. I didn't say talk to them about your healing process because this entails you having to also think about your sickness! For your mind sickness and healing are two sides of the same coin. Your thoughts are energy, mental energy. When you take those thoughts and verbalize them through the power of your speech you have now given those thoughts your life force energy through the process of speaking about them. You will now attract the object of those thoughts. Energy flows where consciousness goes!

What I am talking about here is using your creative thought process to create good health and well being. You see mankind has the power to create and we do this through the power of our thoughts and our visualizations. You are a part of this human race therefore you also have the ability to create! What I would like to do is impregnate your mind with this fact–you are the creator of your own reality. And you manifest this reality through the power of your thoughts, and this includes a healthy body! You are already quite competent in doing this; however for most people this process runs on auto-pilot outside of their awareness. However with a little effort you can become conscious of this process by observing your thoughts and how they make you feel. By doing so you are consciously sending a message to your body that you want it to repair itself! Also that the two of you are on the same page and the same team, and you will do whatever it takes to help it repair itself! However you must remember that anything of true value is worth working for. If you don't give up on yourself and stay true to your goal a healthy body is your birth right. Remember your sickness did not manifest overnight, it took some time to develop, so be patient and kind to yourself especially if it takes a little time for you to really understand this process. We are on a journey of self discovery. Discover the divinity of your true self, because that is healing in and of itself. Step into your power and become the magnificent being that you are meant to be. Good health is your Divine inheritance if you truly want it to be!

Chapter 4 – The Power of Your Beliefs

There was a monastery during medieval times I believe it was located in France. As the story goes, this monastery had the bones of a saint that had died. On certain days of the year the monastery put the bones of the saint on display. Sick people from all over the countryside would flock to this monastery to view the bones of this Saint. People came in great numbers to see these bones and many of those who came were healed of their illness.

This was a mutually beneficial situation for both the sick people and the monks of the monastery. However one night the monastery was broken into and a thief stole the bones of the saint. This was a cause for great concern amongst the monks because the following morning the bones were to be put on display. The monks reported to the head Abbot what had taken place.

The head Abbot decided to dig up some bones from the graveyard in the rear of the monastery and place them on display as the bones of the saint. As usual, the sick flock to the site to view the bones and many of them were healed! The head abbot was totally amazed by this. How could this be he thought? These are not the bones of the saint, how could these healings have happen? Many of the faithful endure great hardships on their journey to this monastery to view these bones with absolute faith that they were going to be healed. The head abbot concluded that the healing power was not in the bones but in the faith of the sick people themselves!

This perhaps is the first documented case of people being healed using a placebo! Today we have many documented cases of people being healed with a placebo. Case studies have been performed with HIV patients where some were given the drug AZT and other a sugar pill. All the patients were told that they were being given the drug AZT. Yet the reality was half of the group was given the drug AZT and the other half a sugar pill. Some HIV patients had results with the drug AZT, and some of them had results with a sugar pill! Let's look at the group that had results with a sugar pill. These people were given no actual medication at all, yet they began to recover.

What do you think expedited the healing process for them? These people believed that they were being given the drug AZT. This drug is very expensive and was out of the price range of some of these patients. These patients believe that the drug AZT would heal them if only they could afford pay for it! Upon being told that they were given the drug AZT free of charge the conscious mind gave the metal body a signal that all was well, and it was time to heal. Also upon receiving a sugar pill, thinking that this was the drug AZT, they became very happy because they were receiving a drug that they could not afford to pay for! This completely infused the emotional body with hope and faith. When the mental body and the emotional body work in tandem with faith healing occurs. The human power of belief is a force that no sickness can stand up to! It worked for the sick people in medieval times that went to the monastery. It worked for the HIV patients. It will work for you today, if you have the courage to use it!

At this point I hope you can understand how the power of the beliefs that were held in the mind of the HIV patients who were given a placebo and the sick people who went to the monastery to view the bone's of the saint, were of paramount importance in their healing process! I cannot stress enough the importance of power your beliefs. This issue is absolutely critical to the success or failure of your healing process!

Your body is your best friend, it is doing everything in its power to keep you alive and healthy; it is one of the most miraculous healing apparatus in the world. It is a self-healing mechanism!

How do you treat your best friend? I'm not talking about your best friend John or Mary, you must treat them well otherwise they will no longer maintain a friendship with you. If you mistreat or abuse them they will tell you where you can go! Your body does not have this luxury, it is stuck with you and you are stuck with it. Again I ask you, how are you treating your best friend? Your body accepts you unconditionally! Do you accept your body? Do you beat the crap out of your body or do you treat it with love and kindness? Some of us live a very busy life and are constantly on the go and the daily grind can be relentless sometimes. We go, go, go, and push our body to the breaking point. Then we are shocked when our body breaks down and becomes sick! We feed our bodies toxic thoughts, toxic emotions and toxic foods. Yet if our best friend, John or Mary was to come to our home for dinner, we would feed them with fine and healthy food and drink. It's all about common sense people, and common sense healing! Our bodies are desperately trying to do everything in their power to keep us alive and healthy. Are you working with your body or are you working against it, only you can honestly answer this question! How are you treating your best friend?

My beliefs are thoughts that I hold in my mind and believe to be true. But the reality of the fact is, just because I believe something and hold that belief in my mind does not make it true! There was a time in our history that we called the dark ages. In this particular time of our history, our ancestors believed that the earth was flat and if you were on a ship sailing on the ocean, you had to be very careful that you did not sail off the edge of the earth! Today this disbelief is totally ridiculous. First of all our scientists have proven and we understand that the earth is not flat at all; it is round or spherical to be more correct. Yet our ancestors believe that if they were on a ship at sea that the navigator of the ship held their life in his hands because he was keeping them from sailing off the edge of the earth! That belief today seems absolutely ridiculous–but it wasn't for our ancestors. Our ancestors experienced fear, and even terror at the thought of sailing off the edge of the earth. This is an indication of the power of belief! My question to you is what do you believe about yourself, your body and your illness? If you have no answer to this question then you have cast your fate to wind and the success of your healing process is like a toss of the dice, they may give you a seven or turn up craps! This is what I mean, when I talk about mental hygiene. You must journey inside your mind and take a good look at what's going on in there. How do your thoughts make you feel? What are your thoughts in relation to your body? Are the thoughts that you are experiencing in your mind so toxic that they cause you to feel bad?

Remember that your body must contend with all this and your thoughts could be so toxic that the emotions that they generate, could also be so negative that your body's immune system could be affected by them! How do you feel about your disease? Do you see it as a death sentence, or as an opportunity of self–discovery? Because if you see yourself on a journey of self–discovery then you can say to yourself what is the sickness trying to teach me? The point I am trying to make here is that you and your body are involved in the dance of life, and your body is your best friend! An important part of maintaining a healthy friendship is to understand your friend and your friend needs! By doing this you maintain a harmonic relationship between you and your best friend. Have a harmonic relationship between your thoughts and your emotions and your body will benefit. Just use your common sense this is what common sense healing is all about!

It has been previously stated that your body is a self-healing mechanism. Your body has consciousness and naturally wants to resonate with health and well-being. The self-healing mechanism of the body is located within the subconscious mind. It performs a myriad of task without you having to spend any conscious energy thinking about them. This is one of the main reasons why I consider my body my best friend. However the subconscious mind is not the only seat of healing within our body. This power to heal is also located within our conscious mind and we can activate its power through our conscious intent! However your belief system plays a critical role in your being able to tap into this power. Remember the people who went to the monastery in France to view the bones of the Saint. Even though the bones of the Saint were no longer there they were still healed by the power of their belief and their faith. Or the HIV patients who were given the sugar pills and believed that they were being given the drug AZT, they were also healed! You can use the power of your belief system to tap into the self-healing power of your body! It is a practical reality that is available to all human beings, and this includes you! I speak to you from a practical experience. I have tap into this power and activated it within my own consciousness, and by doing so today I am able to heal myself and heal others. You have the capability of doing this also. Your belief system plays a critical role in this process. Let me expand on this. There was a time when I was a young boy, when I was trying to learn how to ride a bicycle.

Although I saw other children riding bicycles without any problem I did not believe that I could do that myself. However I did not stop trying and eventually I was able to overcome this belief and today I am quite capable of riding a bicycle. There probably was a time in your life when you like me did not know how to drive a car. We were able to overcome the fear and negative beliefs that we had concerning this process, and today we are quite capable of driving an automobile. Your capability to tap into yourself-healing consciousness is contingent on your beliefs. There is absolutely no doubt in my mind that just like you were able to learn how to ride a bicycle and learn how to drive a car, you are also able to learn how to heal yourself! This is not a gift that Source-Energy has only given to a selected few. We are all children of that "Energy" and this gift has been given to each and every one of us, and this includes you! Rejoice my friend; help is on its way to you, because source energy has guided you to this book. The things that we truly need in life we attract or they find a way to come into our life.

Source Energy has heard you request because you are now holding this book in your hands. It is time for you to move up to the next to the next level of energy in your evolutionary growth process. At this next level it's all about you discovering the power that is within you; you can and will be able to heal yourself! Know this, understand this, believe this, and have the faith that the Source-Energy within you will manifest the knowledge of how to unleash this healing process within your life today, because you are worthy and you deserve it! There is a love inside of you that is so beautiful and so powerful, and this love heals all illness. Allow the illness that you have to teach you exactly what you are doing and how you may be blocking your healing process. By embracing your sickness you will embrace your power! By doing so you will tap into the love that resides within you and you and your sickness can dance into healing, good health, and into unlimited joy!

Please do not see your disease as damnation, but as an opportunity to learn and discover more about who you truly are. And discovering who you truly are is a blessing from the Almighty!

I have observed something most remarkable when I look at children. I noticed they have an instinctive power to heal themselves. Most parents have noticed that whenever their child is in pain, they have a natural tendency to place their hands on whatever part of the body hurts them! If they have a stomach pain, they place their hands on their stomach. If they have a toothache, they place their hands on their mouth, and if they fall and hurt their knee, they will instinctively place their hands on their knee. No one has to tell them to do this, they do it automatically! Children are not removed from the innate capability to heal themselves. They instinctively place their hands on any area that is in pain, and by doing so, they are sending healing energy into that area! They may not be consciously aware of it, but instinctively, they are healing themselves. I will take this a step further if a child falls down and hurts itself it will immediately run to the mother for comfort. The mother will comfort that child and the child well ask mommy to kiss it and make it well! Before that the child is extremely stressed out but the moment the mother kisses that area that is in pain the child immediately calms down. This is indicative of the innate healing power of belief within the child and all of us! The mother may dismiss this as mere child play but if we stop to look at the results the mother could very well learn something from her child! Because that child's belief system is serving it very well and we all started out in this life as children. The mother probably believes she must go to the doctor to get better while the child only has to go to mommy! If the mother could encourage the child to place his or her hands on any area of their body that is in pain she would be reinforcing the natural healing capabilities within her own child! She could come home after a hard day perhaps with a tension headache and say to her child would you like to help mommy heal her headache? Then ask her child to place his or her hands on the affected area and she could be pleasantly surprised at the results! Even if her headache doesn't go away completely she will be reinforcing the belief in her child's capacity to heal itself and others. All human beings have this natural gift! The children are only doing what comes perfectly natural to them by placing their hands on themselves. You are probably asking to yourself, what does this have to do with me, I am not a child. This is true, but you like that child still have access to your own healing capability. Although you may be disconnected from that capability, you do in fact still have it!

I have discovered for myself one of the important processes of my recovery was to make it very clear what I wanted from my body and my life. Be totally clear on exactly what you want, the clearer the better. It has been my experience that there is a power that vibrates within all living things and gives life. If a person just allows themselves to be in a simple state of awareness they can see the manifestations of this power everywhere. The power of life is seeking to manifest itself through you also! There is a divine harmony that resonates throughout this universe, and you are part of this divine resonation whether you realize it or not! The seasons know exactly when to change winter gives way to spring, spring gives way to summer, summer to fall and fall gives way to winter, they never forget and always work in perfect harmony year after year. There is a divine power that has created this process. This divine power has also created you and me also. This divine power is most definitely aware of you! This power also makes itself available to us to offer guidance. However, you and I have been given free will; it is our option to choose or not choose to seek that guidance and act upon it!

After trying everything to overcome my Liver disease, I was right back where I started. It was then I realized I needed all the help I could get. I should like to remind you at this point that my doctors had given up on me. I obviously could not look towards the doctors for help, nevertheless I was still in desperate need of help, but who could I ask? Where was I to look to find guidance? After wrestling with these questions for quite some time I decided it was time to talk to "Source Energy". Who better to help me than the very power that gives life itself, the power that created all of us? If I was going to get involved in a business venture, I would seek help from those who had a proven track record of success. You may be asking yourself what does this have to do with healing? If you are asking yourself this question you have an analytical mind. If you have an analytical mind you are using the power of your brain, and there are some things that go beyond the scope of the brain's power to comprehend! The power of Source-Energy and your connection to that power is one of those things. There are many realities that exist beyond our five senses. Our spiritual reality is one of those realities. I know I am here on a journey of self discovery to discover the divinity that resides in me. Yet there I was at a dead end on my healing journey, with thoughts of death trying to seduce me! Yet for the life of me I could not understand my hesitation in looking towards Source-Energy for help. As a matter of fact it had become quite clear to me that the only power that could in fact help me at this point in time was in fact "Source Energy".

I knew I was going to have to ask for this help, but I was afraid to ask. I then had to ask myself, what exactly was I afraid of? The answer was not being worthy! That response seem so foolish to me today, because today I know we are all worthy of love-each and every one of us, this includes you also! I may not have been worthy in the eyes of my stepfather, or even in my own eyes for that matter, but in the eyes of Source-Energy I am a child of the Divine who is absolutely 100% worthy of all blessings, just like you! So one night after my meditation I decided to sit back and have a talk with that "Source Energy". I was going to see if I could enlist the help of the one who bestows life and good health to all of its children, "Source Energy"!

Chapter 5 – The Mental Body

I as a human being have two modes of thinking, rational and intuitive thinking. Rational thinking is a product of the mind. Intuitive thinking is a product of the emotions. In this chapter I would like to address the rational thinking process as it related to my healing. I shall use the term mental body to refer to the content of thoughts, thought processes and the results they produce. In order to understand and overcome my disease, I needed to better understand the workings of my own mind. I had been traumatized as a young boy. As a result of this my thinking process was flawed and I knew it! I could not afford psychoanalytic therapy so I was going to have to help myself. It is said that the journey of 1000 miles begins with the first step. My first step would be to believe in myself, to believe that I could be healed. My second step would be to instill within my own mind the fact that I was worthy of being healed! I decided that I was going to continue to educate myself. I became a voracious reader. I would seek anything that would bring me a better insight into the workings of my mind. I needed to understand why my thinking process was the way it was if I was going to be able to change it. I knew that the child that resides within me had a broken heart from all the abuse we suffered together. Also that it was of

73

paramount importance to heal this broken heart if I was going to heal my body.

Although I had been abused at a very young age physically, mentally and emotionally, I knew I was very intelligent! This was my intelligence and no one could take it from me, not even my step father! However I knew that my mind and my emotions and I were not working together, we were not on the same page. If I was going to heal my body this would have to change and I knew it!

I decided that I was going to monitor my thoughts. I was not going to try to control them, just watch my thought process as it plays out so to speak. It became very clear to me quite early on that my thoughts were constantly attacking me. This placed in conflict with my own mind! This is a conflict that I had absolutely no way of winning. I began to realize the more these attacks took place, the less energy I had. And the voice that was talking to me inside my head was the voice of my stepfather, who at that time was dead over a decade. Although this man was dead over 10 years he was still causing me to suffer! Please understand what I am trying to say here, I am not blaming my step-father for my disease; I take full responsibility for it. It is my disease, I own it, and it belongs to me! I began to realize that the root cause of my trauma started around the age of 5 years old. After having it beaten into me that I was worthless and not a good son, my mind took this to be true! After all my parents were telling me this and my 5 year old mind believe it. I was not conscious of this belief back then because it was in my subconscious mind! This belief was like a demon lurking in the shadows of my mind. I would face this demon that was blocking my healing process, because my life depended on it! I was going to heal my body and my meditations offered great relief in relaxing my mind to help bring this healing about. However my approach to my healing process would be different from most people. I was not going to a doctor placing all the responsibility of my getting better on the doctor's shoulders. I was not going to make it the doctor's responsible to fix me-that was my job! The doctors only work with the physical body. I would be the "Holistic Doctor" of my own consciousness! Once the mind has been heal the body will follow, I am a firm believer in this.

As I began to look inside of my mind I started to see the content of thoughts within my mental body. I saw low self–esteem, lack of self-worth, and a belief that I could not be like other people; I was different because I was flawed! And as long as I believed this, this was to be my reality! I began to confront myself and started to ask myself when situations arose that brought up these feelings, why do I believe this? Slowly going through this process I was able to discover the root causes of these beliefs. This was my first step towards discovering my own power. Because once you become aware of something then you can change it. Self awareness is the key! This process requires intestinal fortitude however. You must be willing to face your demons so to speak if you are not, you will not receive the many great benefits this process can help you manifest in your life. You must be willing to face your pain, take possession of it and own it! If you are not willing to do this you are better off leaving this pain buried. I believe that if I am going to suffer then it is going to be for the right reasons! Growing pain is perfectly OK with me because I know when I am experiencing growing pain at that point I am and evolving in consciousness and I am growing. The fear and pain that comes from running away from me, I will not tolerate because I cannot run away from myself; I already try that and it didn't work for me.

I had to make these choices concerning my healing process, as you must you make yours also. Time has proven me to be right because today I am 100% Hepatitis free. The virus is not dormant; it isn't in remission; it is gone! This can be your reality also if you willing to pay the price for your recovery.

You may be thinking to yourself, I was not abused like this guy. This stuff does not apply to me. I respond by saying to you if you are ill and your body is not recovering then in some way you are blocking your bodies self-healing process. You probably not doing it intentionally, but never the less in some way either mentally or emotionally you are blocking the self-healing process of your body! I speak from personal experience; I had blocked my healing process for years! However this did not mean that I couldn't change it, I did it and so can you!

I have discovered that for me the two most important factors in my healing process were my thoughts and my beliefs. I will take this a step further and say my thoughts and beliefs are the most important things in the conscious development of my attitude toward my body and its healing process. The key word here is conscious development because with conscious development you learn to set forth your intent! Your intent sends instructions to your body. What are your intentions for your body? If the conscious intent of the mental body is to heal, then your mental energy will give instructions to your body to heal, and your body will act on these instructions. This mental energy stuff should not be taken lightly, because it is quite real and a very powerful tool in the healing process! The mind is the builder of good health but it can also be the builder disease. Most of this process of the mind goes on outside of the conscious awareness of most people. With a little effort you can become conscious of this process. You will begin to realize that your thoughts affect your emotions and these emotions affect your body. The content of your thoughts could be healthy and promote healing or it can be detrimental to you and promote sickness or even death!

It is all about your intention, what do you want for yourself, what do you intend for your body? This is really basically what common sense healing is all about! I remained sick for very long time because I overlook the obvious! You do not have to make the same mistake that I did. Focus your conscious awareness on the content of thoughts. By doing this you will realize how the thoughts you have are making you feel. And consequently you will make the connection between your mental body and your emotional body! This will catapult you forward in your healing process. Your thoughts can reveal to you how you truly feel about yourself and your body. It is of paramount importance for you to understand this! When I began to understand how I truly felt about my body I was shocked. There were so many things about my body I disliked or even hated. I wasn't happy with my hair and I was displeased with my weight and angry that my body was susceptible to asthma attacks. These were just a few things I disliked about my body; I had a long list back then. Yet today I am fully aware of the fact that I have no better friend in this life than my body. It does absolutely everything in its power to keep me alive and healthy in spite of what I did to it. Now that's a friend!

It would be of great benefit to you to discover how you feel and the type of relationship you have with your body. However this should be done with great love and kindness and without any judgment because whatever the relationship with your body and the feelings you have about it are; once you become conscious and aware of that relationship then you can make changes. The greater portion of my healing process was all about overcoming the self limitations that I placed on myself by the power of my limiting thoughts! You can also do this, however it would benefit you greatly to be kind to yourself. Treat yourself with the same love and kindness that you would like to receive from others. We must learn to love ourselves if we are going to heal. This is something only you can teach yourself. I know of no college curriculum that has a course to teach you how to love yourself. If you have not learned this skill from your parents, it doesn't mean that you must go through life without it. Once I began to realize that the power of the divine vibrated within my being, I began to understand that there was nothing I could not do!

What I am attempting to do here is to help you set a mental foundation which will assist you to promote your own healing. This is what I called mental hygiene, to be able to place your mind on the thoughts that make you feel good and promote healing, and remove your focus from all thoughts that are toxic to your body and to your healing process! You and I have the power to choose what we think about. There is power in this freedom of choice. And no one can choose for you. You and I are co; creators with Source Energy, and we create through the power of thought! When I finally got this – really understood it, it was so very liberating for me. I no longer had to be the victim of my past or my thoughts, and neither do you! Tap into the power of your healing mind; make it one of your greatest assets because it is; but you must discover this for yourself to make it a reality in your life!

The power of your mind is unlimited and when it works in tandem with your emotions you become the powerful creator that you were meant to be!

I want to expand on the concept mental hygiene a bit more here. Most people when they wake up the first thing they do is jump into the shower to clean their body. Physical hygiene is given a high priority but mental hygiene falls fairly low on the list of most people's priorities. Mental and emotional hygiene are equally as important as physical hygiene, however they are usually neglected! It may seem that I am stating the obvious here, however most people have a tendency of overlooking the obvious. I was guilty of this fact for many years of my life! When I finally understood this concept of mental hygiene, it hit me like a ton of bricks. The way I was spoken to as a young child was very abusive, and especially by my step father who was extremely abusive, mentally, emotionally and physically. Whenever I've made a mistake I was called dumb or stupid. The only reason I mention this point here is because we all have an internal dialogue with ourselves, and the voice that talks to you inside your head is usually the voice of your parents or caregivers. I realized I had internalized my stepfather's abusive way of communicating with myself! It was the voice of my internal dialog within me and it was very negative and very abrasive. It had been imprinted upon me at a very young age. I could even hear the harsh tone of my stepfather's voice inside my head! He had inflicted a great deal of abuse upon me as a child. Now I could see that because he was imprinted within my subconscious as a result I was now inflicting that same kind of abuse upon myself! This was totally unacceptable. But now that I had become aware that this process was going on within my own head, I decided to do something about it.

I use to believe that I had absolutely no control over my thought process.

Scientists say that the average person has anywhere from up to 50,000 thoughts a day! I will speak form my own experience. I have absolutely no control over the incoming thought process but what I do have control of is the thoughts

I choose to place my focus on! This is very important because now I have the power of choice. This means I do not have to be a victim or allow myself to be overwhelmed by my incoming thoughts. In performing my mental hygiene the most important thing I have to be aware of are the content of my thoughts. At that point in time some of them are very beautiful thoughts that promote health and well being, while others were toxic and only promote sickness. I have the power to choose where I place my focus and attention. This means I have the power to choose thoughts that promote health and well-being. By doing so I am performing my mental hygiene! It's all about me using my common sense and understanding that this is a process that the doctors cannot do for me! Using my commonsense has brought me to the understanding of commonsense healing and how it works. It actually is very simple and not complicated at all. It can be done by anyone; it just requires a little work to bring your mind into the awareness of what you are thinking. There is only one prerequisite, you must be willing to go within your mind and honestly see how you are thinking and how those thoughts are making you feel! And if you are willing to do this the odds are that you can overcome your illness. Remember that your body is a self-healing mechanism and has great intelligence but you must nourish it and take care of it. You must remember as I had to that your mental energy is a reflection of your thoughts. Also the fact that these thoughts have an impact on your emotional body which constitutes the way you feel. We are not just physical beings we are mental and emotional beings also. When we have these aspects of ourselves, the physical, mental, and emotional working in harmony good health is the result.

The question some of you may be asking yourself now is how does one become aware of their thoughts? An excellent way of doing this is to just be aware of what you are feeling, because emotion is generated by thought. However if you come from an abusive background you may have been led to believe like I was, that your feelings are not important. Nothing could be further from the truth! It is of paramount importance that you feel good!

When you feel good your energy has a harmonious flow. This places you in harmony with yourself and your body. Allowing your body to do what it naturally wants to do and that is to heal itself! Let me state here that the mental body and emotional body are heads and tails of the same coin. They work in tandem whether you are conscious of that fact or not. Many of us have worked very hard repressing our thoughts and emotions because we have found them to be very painful. However by doing this over long periods of time you can manifest disease in your body. If you have done this and you have manifest a disease in your body, your body is telling you it can no longer tolerate the content of the repressed emotion and the toxic thoughts that you are feeding it!

Your body is constantly communicating with you all the time. It is our job to learn how to communicate with and learn the language with which our body speaks to us. This is something that you already instinctively know how to do. You just need to allow the body wisdom that is in your heart to enter your mind! Your body is intelligent and naturally wants to resonate with health and well-being. Your body has the gift of intuitive intelligence and is doing everything in its power to keep you alive and healthy. However your physical body listens to and follows the commands that it is given by the body of thoughts that are contain in your mental body [conscious mind]. If the content of thoughts that are contained in your mental body is toxic then the physical body will suffer, break down and eventually get sick. I cannot overstate the importance and power of your thoughts! They can be the building blocks to excellent health or your thoughts can bring you disease! Only you can monitor the thought process that takes place in your mental body no one else can do it for you. However once you get the hang of it is very easy to do. I am attempting to lay down a foundation for you to understand how you can take charge of your mind so that you may heal your body. I want you to understand that you are a co; creator which source energy and you can create good health for yourself if you so desire!

Chapter 6 – The Emotional Body

At this point I would like to address the subject of the emotional body and its contents. The content of my emotional body is the result of the body of thoughts that are contained within my mind. Let me clarify what I mean here. I have a friend named Adrienne. Adrienne is a very happy person with a great sense of humor; it is a pleasure to be around her. If I am feeling down it always makes me feel better just to be around her. She is what I like to call a happy camper because the overall content of her emotional body is happiness. I also know a man named Simon. He is always angry and always upset about something. My nickname for him is anger man. The point I'm trying to make here is your overall disposition is a reflection of the content of your emotional body which is in turn is a result of the content of your thoughts! Today at this point in my life the overall content of my emotional body is positivity and easy-goingness. However this was not always the case. I was once like my friend Simon, I was also anger man! There is nothing wrong with being angry; anger is one of the basic emotions and we all get angry from time to time. But if anger is the predominant emotion in your emotional body, then you are living your life out of anger. Sustained anger over long periods of time becomes toxic to your body and will break down your immune system and can cause you to be prone to disease! When I was living my life out of the emotion of anger I would find reasons to justify me being angry. By doing that I was giving myself permission to be angry, and by saying to myself it was okay to in fact be in angry. Even though I was justifying my anger it was still toxic to my body! Eventually I finally became conscious of this situation. Once I became conscious of this situation my conscious mind gave me a direction that it was time to do something about it! The first thing I decided to do was find the cause of this anger and the reasons for the behavior that caused me to justify it! I discovered that the root cause of this anger was the victimization and the trauma that I had suffered by the abuse that was inflicted upon me by my stepfather. This was not at all hard to discover. However it took a little more time to discover the reasons for justifying the anger.

This required some soul-searching. I needed to be brutally honest with myself. I was searching for the truth not excuses!

I realize that my subconscious mind would not manifest the true reasons for my behavior until I was honestly ready to receive those answers! After a short period of time I knew I was ready to receive these answers because they manifested in my conscious mind. Living my life from anger allowed me to play the role of the victim! Justifying my anger was a process that I had learned unconsciously from my step father-he also lived his life out of anger and he also played the role of victim! This was something that was very hard for me to swallow because I did not like this man and I did not want to be anything thing like him! I was beginning to understand that his behavior had been imprinted upon me very deeply. Like it or not our parents and caregivers behavior are imprinted upon us! Now that I was conscious of this I did not have to tolerate this behavior within myself any more. I now had a choice and my choice was to do something about it.

The quantity of anger that had manifested in my life was overwhelming. I did not run away from this anger, I took responsibility for it and made my own! I also noticed when I was going through my illness that I had to be aware of how I was behaving. When I was experiencing my disease, I saw myself behaving in such a way that really was not beneficial to my healing process. Because of the abuse I received growing up I was desperate for love in my life. I began to notice that I would talk to anyone who would listen to me about my disease! Meditation helped me become conscious that I was doing this. Once I became conscious of this behavior I could ask myself the question, why am I doing this? What I became aware of was that I was looking for sympathy-yes sympathy! This was a way that my inner child who was living within was trying to get love. However by behaving in this way I was operating out of the victim mode. Anyone who gave me sympathy was reinforcing within me the position I had unconsciously taken of seeing myself as a victim! As long as I would allow this to continue this I would remain a victim and could not heal!

When this behavior manifested in my consciousness it showed me that I was disconnected from my inner child. I was forcing my inner child to settle for sympathy, but what it really wanted was love! I was disconnected from my inner child and consequently I was not giving him love! As a result here I was a grown man going through life looking for sympathy! This behavior also kept me focused on my illness instead of my healing. At that point in my life I now understood that whatever I focused my attention on I was going to attract. And I wanted to attract healing not sickness. This behavior of going through life looking for sympathy could no longer be tolerated! In order to change this behavior I was going to have to listen to the voice of my inner child. No one could give him love but me, and he really wanted love not sympathy!

Slowly but surely my emotional body was revealing its content to me. I was beginning to understand why I was so afraid. That little five-year-old boy that had been traumatized was living inside of me and he was still terrified! I needed to address the emotional issues that had been created as a result of the trauma we suffered together. At that time in my life all this was a bit overwhelming for me. So I decided to proceed down this path slowly taking it one step at a time. I decided that I was going to set up a dialogue between me and this five-year-old boy that resides within me. The first thing I decided to do was to give him a name; I decided to call him Junior the name he was called when we were growing up. And the next thing I decided to do was to create a safe zone, so whenever we would have a conversation he would feel absolutely safe and protected! To many of you it may seem like I have gone off the deep end here! However my attitude was that I was going to heal myself by any means necessary and this was absolutely necessary; besides I had nothing to lose by trying! So one morning after meditation I decided to go into the living room. I took a chair for the kitchen table and put it in the living room near the couch. I sat quietly on the couch for a moment and then began to visualize that little 5 year old boy who was a manifestation of my past. I felt his presence instantly! Then I ask Junior if he would like to share anything with me. He responded yes, that he would like to talk to me. I asked him if he would like to come out and sit on the kitchen chair and he said yes he would. At that very moment I felt a warm sensation in the center of my heart that was very comforting. I looked at the kitchen chair and began to speak just like Junior was sitting right there. I told him that he had absolutely nothing to worry about anymore because I was there for him and I was going to protect him from this moment on! Upon speaking these words out loud it was as if a great weight had been lifted off my shoulders. I actually began to feel energy coming from the kitchen chair, coming to me. I asked Junior if there was anything that he wanted me to do for him. He asked me if I would allow him to sit on my lap and if I would hold him. My response was yes I would. I began to feel a tingling sensation in my lap and also around my neck. It felt exactly like I was holding a five-year-old child in my lap who had placed his arms around my neck. My words could never express how good this felt! At that moment I knew I'd taken a traumatized part of myself and was acknowledging it by giving it comfort, and love! What I felt at that moment was a contentment that was truly uplifting. Slowly but surely I was finally becoming whole. After that first session between Junior and me the level of my anger drop significantly! I had now established a dialogue with my inner child and as a result I had also opened a deeper dialogue with my emotional body which is part of my subconscious mind!

I had always wanted love in my life but I did not know how to love myself. Life through my disease was now teaching me how to do just that! Yes that's right my disease was teaching me some valuable lessons and I was open to learn them all. By acknowledging my inner child I was now accepting a part of me that had been repressed and disowned for many years. By doing this I was saying yes to life, yes to my body and yes to my healing process! I was learning to listen to the intuitive voice that was coming from my higher self. We all are in possession of divine knowledge, each and every one of us; we just need to learn how to access it. Meditation has given me the key to open the door to my higher self, and access that higher knowledge. The first thing that was on the agenda for my higher self and I was to heal this body. I was now getting the assistance of the best doctor in the universe, my higher self! There was absolutely no doubt within me that I would overcome this disease! I believed that right down to the core of my very being, because I was doing exactly what the great Socrates said 2500 years ago " Know Thyself ", and this self knowledge was giving me the power to heal!

I have said that the thoughts that you allowed to occupy your mind stream are of the utmost importance to your body. Why is this so, because the thoughts that you allow to occupy your mind stream will generate feelings in your emotional body. These feelings can move about throughout various places in your physical body. Sometimes your thoughts can generate fear and you can feel that fear in the pit of your stomach! If you feel that the one you love is cheating on you, you will feel the pain in your heart! All of us have had this experience on one level or another. This is not to be taken lightly, because it is of the utmost importance to your emotional hygiene. It is at that moment that your physical body is communicating with you! Your body is telling you that the thoughts that you are allowing to occupy your mind stream are generating emotions that are causing it pain and suffering! Please listen to your best friend! At this point, your physical body is talking to you but are you listening? This is what I mean when I say you must learn the language of your body!

All of us have gone to school at one time or another and we have been taught many things, but none of us have been taught how to listen to our bodies! Our bodies do talk to us in its own language all the time. You must learn and understand the language of your own body, especially if your body is sick and you want to restore it back to good health! This is not as difficult as it may sound. Actually it is quite simple. All it takes is a shift in conscious awareness and a willingness to understand why you feel the way that you do. I repeat the words of that great master Socrates once again; "*Know Thyself*". However people spend a great deal of time, money, and energy on a daily basis trying to escape what they feel! By acting in this manner they are saying no to life and yes to death! You cannot escape from your feelings they are intertwined with the essence of your very being! We came to earth school because we are on a journey of self-discovery. The magnificent being that you are is greater and more powerful than any negative emotion you could ever have! I know this to be true from my own experience. You must discover this for yourself and by doing so you can help your body heal. Your precious human body is doing everything in its power to keep you alive and healthy; are you doing everything in your power to help it help you? Step up to the plate and become a partner with your body and watch the magic unfold! You can do it! You can heal yourself! You can say yes to your life! I am not just talking the talk, I am walking the walk; according to the doctors, by all rights I should be dead now! Yet here I sit today talking to you through this book. My Liver Disease is not dormant, it is not in remission-it is gone! But there is a price I had to pay. I had looked into my mind and see the thoughts that were in my mental body. I had to see what emotions those thoughts were generating in my emotional body and how my physical body was responding to those thoughts. There is a price to pay for your recovery and this is a price that you cannot pay with cash. You can only pay this price with love and courage! Please make this investment in yourself and your healing process and dare to become the magnificent human being you were meant to be!

Chapter 7 - Activating the Healing Mindset

The healing mindset is not a tangible thing, yet it is nonetheless very real. Everyone has access to their own healing mindset, whether they realize it or not. Your overall thoughts and feelings, and the actions that you take as a result of those feelings are indicative of the healing mindset you posses!

Introspection and self-awareness is the key here. The introspective factor is you going inside to honestly take a look at the thoughts in your mind. There should be no judgment here; you must allow yourself to be okay with whatever your thoughts are! Judgment at this point may lead you to self sabotage, and you don't want to do that. What was very helpful for me was adopting an attitude of watching with curiosity, like a person who brings home a new puppy dog and just watches it to see how it behaves. There is no judgment there, just a curiosity to see how your mind behaves. Watch with kindness and affection just like you were watching your puppy to get to know it better. Keep a lighthearted attitude and just observe your thoughts without any judgment. Are your thoughts angry thoughts, sad thoughts or thoughts of hopelessness? Are you thinking to yourself, why did this have to happen to me? And whatever you are thinking is perfectly okay, just become aware of your thinking process. However this may take a little time in the beginning so do not beat yourself up if you don't get it right away. You see beating yourself up is just another form of self punishment and will only attract more sickness, it's just common sense. You must make peace with where you are right now! This is the first step of stepping into your healing consciousness. And when you do this you are now on the path to conscious awareness of your mental body. Now your healing journey has begun in earnest, because now you are becoming aware of and stepping onto the path of understanding your mental body! Congratulations you are now stepping into your power and stepping into your power is the first step in returning your body back wholeness and good health. Now because you are monitoring the thoughts in your mental body, you can take the next step!

Your thoughts generate the emotions that you feel, and the overall state of those emotions I call the emotional body. Do you know someone who is lighthearted and happy most of the time? You may use to term that I use when I refer to them as a happy camper. The term happy camper is indicative of the state their emotional body. What is the state of your emotional body? If you don't know that's okay because you can find out what it is! This is a very easy thing to do. Just look to see how your thoughts make you feel. Again just watch with curiosity, there is no need for judgment here! How do you honestly feel? Not how you think you should feel, but how do you honestly feel? There's no right or wrong here, however you are feeling is perfectly okay, if you allow it to be okay. Be brave and have the courage to allow it to be okay! I know you can do this! You may be thinking to yourself I do not want to do this-this could be painful. My question to you is this; is it more painful than being sick? Only you can be the judge of that! The price you pay for being sick you pay every day of your life as long as you are sick! The price that you pay for you healing is a one-time payment. And when you pay the price of healing which is a onetime payment, good health is the return on your investment. The choice is yours! The doctors cannot do this work for you; they work with your physical body. Only you can activate your healing mindset. Only you can do the work it takes to bring your consciousness into harmony with your mental and emotional body which in turn will assist your physical body in repairing itself! You must work in tandem with your doctor. Help your doctor help you heal. Activate your healing mindset! Discovered the content of your mental and emotional body, then take responsibility for that content-own it! Step into your power and allow the self-healing mechanism that is your body to heal itself! Become your body's best friend. Stop berating yourself because your body is sick. Your body is intelligent, and naturally wants to resonate with health and well-being!

You can trust your body. Your body is magnificent. You are magnificent. Step into your healing mindset and discover the magnificent being that is you. The power of the Divine walks with you! Step out of that mindset of sickness. You owe it to yourself. Open the gates to your healing mindset and step into good health. It is your birth right!

Your healing mindset is like the wand of the magician and when the wand of that healing mindset touches your body magic will happen; one can heal. There is a transformation in the mindset first and then the body takes it cues from that mindset! The transformation from sickness to health is also a process of self discovery-to become aware of you within you! Many people as I did go through life not wanting to face themselves. I did this out fear. But if a person can allow the fear to be there and continue onward courage is the reward and fear must retreat! However fear will regroup and attack you again to probe for a weakness within you. It will attempt to use the power of your mind against you because the fear is a product of the mind! You must be aware of this! Every individual will have a way their mind attacks them. It is good to understand the personality and temperament of your own mind, especially if you are trying to heal your body. But you see most of this knowledge you already have within you, I just want to reconnect you to it. How you may ask? By using your common sense and stepping up into your magnificence. There is wisdom within all living things that wisdom is also within you. For me I had the opportunity to access that wisdom when I open up a dialog with myself. For then I started to become aware my mind, my body and my sprit and they all wanted to live! However they were not working in harmony with one another and this was a contributing factor in to my disease and I knew it. I didn't have to put up with this because through the power of my will I could manifest that harmony that was needed. But there was a price to pay and that was to search within myself and honestly look at what was going on–without any judgment! Once you see what going on, what would you like to do? If you see what going on but you are not sure of what to do, that's okay. You see by observing your mind and emotions and seeing conflict that you want resolved your subconscious mind will now search for options and help you resolve this conflict, you just need to know how to enlist its help.

Many people as I did come to a point in their journey where they hit a wall. When this happen to me I felt overwhelmed; this was because I was reaching the limits of my comfort zone. This feeling usually brings fear, panic and a sense of totally freaking out. This is because you are expanding in consciousness and the limits of the old threshold no longer suffice; so a new threshold must be created at a higher level. However this is an evolutionary growth process to be at this threshold dead end, and it is not a comfortable feeling–but the breakthrough to the next level and the development of a new and greater comfort zone threshold feels out of sight! The point I am trying to make here is that you are embarking on a journey from sickness to health. You will take your body to a state of health and well being and in the process discover that it is your best friend and it is a self-healing mechanism! It is a worthy container for that spark of the Divine that is you!

Understanding the interplay between the conscious and subconscious mind was of great benefit to me in my healing process, as it can also be for you in yours. Do not be intimidated by the terminology conscious and subconscious mind because it will be very easy for you to understand the interplay between the two! I will use an analogy here to make it easy for you to comprehend the information I am giving you now. Let's say your body is a ship a vessel so to speak. The captain of the ship is your "Conscious Mind". The crew of the ship is your "Subconscious Mind". The captain of the ship your "*Conscious Mind*" is the one who commands the ship by giving the orders to the crew. The crew your "*Subconscious Mind*" must follow the commands of the captain and they must do so without question. It is the responsibility of the crew the "*Subconscious Mind*" to maintain and service the ship, your body! The subconscious mind does an excellent job of this and performs a myriad of task outside of your awareness. Such as digesting the food you eat, growing your hair and fingernails and automatically healing you when you hurt yourself. However your subconscious mind must follow the commands of your conscious mind no matter what they are! This is why it is so important to be aware of the content of thoughts within your mental body. You're "*Subconscious Mind*" the crew must act on the commands of the Captain your "*Conscious Mind*" even if those commands produce something you do not want!

Another very important point is that your mind cannot process a negative! If I say to you do not think about a white car what is the first thing that comes into your mind? Most likely it will be a white car even though I told you do not think about a white car. This is so because your mind cannot process a negative! If you think to yourself I do not want to be sick your mind must focus on sickness even though this is what you do not want. As a result of the mind focusing on sickness it will attract sickness! It does so because it cannot process a negative. Also what you focus your mind on, your mind will attract! If the mind has been given the subject of sickness it will focus on sickness and therefore attract sickness! Instead focus on what you really want and that is good health. Use the power of your conscious thought. You have the capability to focus your thoughts on whatever you want. The key is to be clear on what you want and stay focused on that!

Remember that your subconscious mind is responsible for taking care of your body however it must follow the commands given by the captain the conscious mind. Becoming aware of the content of thoughts within your conscious mind will serve you well and will give you the insights you need to see the things you may be doing that may be promoting sickness in your body. Many times you may be committing self sabotage through a part of your thought process. However discovering these insights are very valuable to your healing process and you cannot get these insights from your doctor! You must be the one to look into your own mind to see what you may be doing that might be contributing to your illness. If you are not doing anything to contribute to your illness then that's good. However should you discover that you are doing something to self sabotage, you now have the option to reprogram that particular thought pattern!

Many people believe that they have absolutely no control over their thoughts. This is just not true. You may not have any say in what thoughts come into your mind but you do have control of what thoughts you place your focus on! You might be asking yourself now, how will I know the right thoughts to focus on? You will know based on how those thoughts makes you feel. Good feeling thoughts promote healing! If the body of thoughts you are thinking makes you feel bad, down or depressed a simple shift in your focus can change the way you feel. By doing this you will come to understand how the thoughts in your mental body affect your emotions. And how the content of your emotions affect your feelings and their impact on your physical body! Once you understand this process, the interplay between the mental, emotional and physical bodies, that awareness puts you on the fast track to healing. It has been my experience that by paying attention to the little details one comes to a greater understanding of the big picture! By understanding your thoughts you will come to a better understanding of why you feel the way you do. When this understanding comes into you then you will see the direct impact that those thoughts have on your body. Those details will give you a better understanding of your own big picture as it pertains to your healing process!

Just as a person can be out of touch with their feelings, a person can be out of touch with their body as well! I had been out of touch with my body for years. When a person is out of touch with their body they will usually not realize it until after they become sick. By monitoring the thoughts contained in your mental body and their impact on your emotions and how those emotions make you feel, you will gradually get back in touch with your body if you are in fact out of touch with it. Self awareness is the key here.

Get to know your best friend-your body! By doing so the two of you can work in tandem because your body could use your help to keep you healthy. The idea of your body as your best friend may be just a concept for you now. However I cannot overstate the importance of the dynamics of this relationship and its benefit to your healing! When I became my body best friend I would find the time to listen to what it was trying to communicate to me. It is just common sense! How do you feel when you are ignored? Now ask yourself this question, how do you think your body feels when you ignore it? Here is this magnificent apparatus that allows me to have the gift life and I was ignoring it, my best friend! I would listen to everyone else except my body. I would watch television and listen to all the media hype telling me how I should look and be in this world. I was failing to see the motivation of the sponsors and that was to sell me their products! My body accepts me unconditionally and has done so for my entire life yet I did not accept it! Behaving in this manner was what was keeping me from getting back in touch with my body. This is why I was sick for such a long time. My illness was teaching me how to live in harmony with my body and when I learned this lesson I was finally able to heal! Discover the lessons that your sickness is trying to teach you and you can heal also!

I have worked with people who actually hate their bodies. Ask them what they do not like about their body and they have a long list of things they feel are wrong with their body. I say to you, here and now, the longer the list of things you dislike about your body, the greater the self rejection!

Please understand the point I am trying to make here. If there are things you dislike about your body and you can improve on them by all means do so!

But if you have what you consider a weight problem and the average weight of the men and women on your family tree is 200 lbs. then try to come to terms with this. Why you may ask because if you try to maintain a weight of 110 lbs. and your natural body weight is 200 lbs. you do so at the risk of your own health! This is why so many people gain the weight right back after a diet because the body is readjusting itself to maintain proper balance and health. I had to learn to accept my best friend so I could accept myself. By doing so I was able to see the downfalls that were keeping me in ill health and so will you!

Chapter 8 – The Power of Repressed Emotions

I had a very good friend named Mallory. She had been to see three different doctors about sores she had on her right hand. Although she saw three doctors, and they all gave her three different prescriptions, none of them worked. The sores got much worse, to the point where the skin was beginning to separate, and you could see the meat underneath the skin down to the bone! Needless to say this situation caused her great frustration and was the cause of much concern for her. I stopped by her house to pay her a visit and found her crying at the kitchen table. I was unaware of what was going on with her and ask her what was the matter? She did not answer me and continued sobbing, and she just showed me her hand. I sat at the kitchen table beside her and didn't say anything. I just allowed her to continue to cry. I could see very clearly that she needed to cry, in order to release her some of her anger and frustration. I sat there quietly and allowed her to do just that! She wept very intensely for what seemed to be a very long time.

When she finally finished, she looked at me with a look of frustration and embarrassment and apologize for crying. The intensity of her gut wrenching sobbing had almost brought a tear to my eye!

At that point I stood up from the table, reached out and took her left hand, pulled her close to me and we embraced. We sat down at the table again, and she told me exactly what happened with the doctors. I sat there quietly and just listened. Something she said caught my attention. She told me that she was so angry and upset that she felt like she wanted to cut her hand off! I began to realize that what was going on with her hand was just the tip of the iceberg. I ask if she wanted me to help her and in a moment of anger she lashed out at me. She said Jimmy if the doctors can help me what the hell can you do? At this point I told her Mallory, the doctors are only looking at your body, what if the source of this problem does not lie in your body! Jimmy she said what on earth are you talking about? I said we have been friends for a long time Mallory. Please let me try to help you. At this point she asked me, what do you want me to do? I don't want you to do anything I responded. Just sit here quietly with me for a moment and allow me to give you a reading. I looked at her body, then close my eyes and quietly said a prayer. Instantly, a vision began to manifest in my mind stream. I sat there quietly and watch this vision just like someone sitting in a movie. When the vision was over, I opened my eyes. As I looked at her I could see tears streaming down her face. I said to her Mallory, I have some things to tell to you that are going to be very painful! I am your friend and I care about you very much and you know that. I know that what I have to say can help you a great deal, but I must tell you it's going to be painful! Do I have your permission to share this information with you? She answered yes! Okay, I said, about 12 years ago you had an abortion. The child that you aborted was a girl, and this girl had beautiful blonde curly hair. Whenever you see a girl with blonde curly hair, about 12 years old, you think about the child that you aborted. Then you feel a tremendous amount of guilt, and you tell yourself I murdered my baby! Day after day, month after month, year after year, you have done nothing but swallow this guilt. By doing so you have decreased the healing capability of your immune system! Telling me that you want to cut off your right hand is your way of trying to atone for the guilt that you feel! At this point, she exploded into a gut wrenching weeping. This went on for about 20 minutes. Finally she stopped! I began to talk to her again. And as I did I began to twirl my hair at the ends. I am bald with a shaved head! I did not understand why I was doing that but I couldn't stop myself. I continue to speak with her as I continue to twirl my hair. As I spoke with her, my demeanor and the tone of my voice began to visibly change. I said to her Mallory, when you got pregnant with this child, you were only 16 years old! You were still a child yourself and you were not ready for motherhood. The child that you were carrying was a very special child and you named her Elena. To complete her journey on the earth plane, Elena only needed to experience being in a womb and being loved by you! It was not necessary for her to

111

incarnate on the earth plane and experience all the pain and suffering that we human beings go through. As I am speaking to her, I continue to play with my hair. Mallory God has forgiven you, Elena has forgiven, and now you need to forgive yourself! When I said this to her jaw dropped, oh my God she said, Jimmy your demeanor has changed, your voice has also changed, and you are playing hair that you don't have. When I dream of my Elena, and she speaks to me and the intonation of her voice sounds exactly like the way you're speaking to me now. And she is always twirling her hair with her right hand, just like you are doing right now. My God, my daughter is speaking to me through you! At this point, she began to weep once more, but this time it was very different. The anger, frustration and bitterness had vanished. When she finished crying, she was able to muster up a smile! I don't believe what just happened, she said, it seemed like something out of a movie. I must confess though, I feel much better now!

Mallory there is something that Elena wants you to understand, Einstein proved that energy cannot be created, nor can it be destroyed. There is no greater energy than the power of love! The love between mother and daughter is one of the greatest loves. That bond of love transcends life and death! Mallory's energy had completely shifted and her smile was radiating the entire room. But we were not finished yet there was still the issue of her right hand!

112

Mallory is an active woman, she is not the type of person to sit idly by and watch things happen to her. I needed to give her something to do, something to make her feel like she was actively participating in the healing process of her hand! Mallory I said, this is what Elena would like you to do, purchase a pair of cotton gloves. At night just before you go to bed, wash your hand with soap and water rub it with alcohol and Vaseline, then put the cotton glove on your right hand. Do this for two weeks and your hand will be healed. Mallory called me six days later, her hand was completely healed. This is the power of the emotional body!

What exactly do I mean when I say this is the power of the emotional body? In Mallory's case she got very little results by going to doctors.

Doctors are trained to focus their attention on the symptoms that manifest in the physical body but in Mallory's case the root cause of the problem did not lie in the physical body! The source of the problem was in the mental and emotional bodies. Every time she saw a 12-year-old girl with blonde curly hair her mental process triggered her guilt mechanism. The thoughts in this guilt mechanism were telling her that she had murdered her daughter. She believed this and this created an onslaught of emotions. These emotions in their very nature were toxic and led her to believe that she was unworthy of forgiveness and did not deserve to live! She had repressed these thoughts and emotions for over a decade and it finally reached the point where they could not be repressed any longer! Through her thoughts she had created a belief, that belief created emotions. The body of toxic thoughts that created that belief I call the mental body. The block of emotions that was created as a result of that belief, I refer to as the emotional body.

Mallory would wake up every morning and perform her physical hygiene. She took pride in her appearance and great pride in her body. However her mental hygiene and her emotional hygiene were non-existent! No one and I mean no one can perform your mental or emotional hygiene for you. I'm sure no one will disagree that if you don't keep your body clean you will get sick, this is quite obvious. What may not be as obvious is that if you don't perform your mental and emotional hygiene, the results can be very devastating. Mallory is a prime example of that. Just as no one knows your body better than you do, no one knows your thoughts and feelings better than you do either! What I am suggesting that you do requires courage. Most people are not aware of their thought processes, they just think without paying much attention to the consequences of their thoughts.

People also spend a great amount of time and a great amount of money in trying to escape their thoughts and emotions. However you cannot run away from you! Do your mental and emotional hygiene and your physical body will love you for it. This is how you empower yourself and take control of your healing process. This is the crux of common sense healing!

At this point we come to a very delicate subject, how you view yourself and how you view your body. You may be asking yourself what does this have to do with healing? This has a great deal to do with your healing process because how you view yourself and your body has a very strong influence on the energy that you resonate. There are so many courses and programs today on self-improvement. However there is a point I would like to make to you that is of paramount importance. The self that you are trying to improve upon your true self needs no improvement! Everyday each and every one of us is hit with a barrage of information from the media, most especially women. The media has set an impossible standard of how we should be, how we should act and how we should look! We are constantly being told that the way we are is just not acceptable! Women are constantly being targeted and told that their hair is not acceptable, you should buy this product! That their eyelashes are not acceptable, so what you need to do is buy that product! That they are too fat but if you buy this weight loss product or enroll in that weight loss program then you will be perfect.

Nothing could be further from the truth!

The truth of the matter is you are already perfect! A perfect power has created you and that power has made no mistakes! I'm trying to point these things out to you for very important reason. If you buy into all of this media hype your level of self acceptance decreases! This will have a powerful impact on your mental and emotional states and the thoughts and feelings that you emanate from your energy field. And remember that like energy attracts like energy! If you are putting out a vibration of self rejection what do you think is going to return to you? You will attract people who will reinforce your belief that you are not good enough and these people in turn will reject you! This will cause you to sink deeper and deeper into depression so if you do in fact have a weight problem, this will cause you to seek comfort. You will do so by looking for immediate gratification, usually in food, thereby perpetuating your weight problem! If you're not aware of this there is absolutely nothing you can do about it. It is my hope that by reading these pages you will bring this into your conscious awareness. When that happens you will now have a choice! This means that you can choose thoughts that will create feelings more beneficial to you and your body. Do you actually think that the model on the cover of Vogue magazine really looks like that? The effects of lights and cameras are being used to enhance the way she really looks. After that the photo is taken it is touched up with an air brush. A truly beautiful woman can put on a pair of jeans and a sweatshirt and still look drop dead gorgeous and so can a handsome man.

Our culture tells us that to grow old is a bad thing, yet none of us can stop the aging process! We are hit with an avalanche of so much information that is telling us how we should be, and that the way we are is just not good enough. Please do not buy into any of this media hype! The Source-Energy that has created you has made you incredibly beautiful, even if you don't see yourself as being beautiful; all that means is that you have yet to discover your own beauty! Most of us are familiar with the children's story of the ugly duckling. The little duckling was constantly abuse and rejected by all of the other animals. One day it saw a beautiful formation of swans flying in the sky and thought I wish I could be as beautiful as those swans; having thought that it bowed its head in shame and was at that point that it saw its reflection in the water. The transformation had taken place it had become what it was meant to be-a magnificent swan! Step into the magnificent being that you truly are. Discover your beauty and soar like that swan. You are beautiful, you are magnificent and you are Divine!

There are many different healing modalities that are in use today. Most people go to see a doctor first. However in many cases where the doctors do not produced the desired result, a person may seek out alternative modes of therapy of which there are many. A person might go to see a

117

chiropractor who will apply pressure to and perform spinal manipulation. One could also go to acupuncturist who works with the channels and meridians within the body. There are many faith healers work with the power of prayer. There are also some healers who use the laying on of the hands technique, I personally have learned and develop this technique and have great results with it, and have used it to help many people. I have a friend who also gets very good results with flower remedies. These are just a few of the many healing techniques that are available for one to try. The point I would make here is that if you are seeking alternative medical treatment you must do your homework! Different people get different results with different modalities!

Human beings are a manifestation of divine energy. This divine energy flows through and resonates throughout their entire body. This divine energy also constitutes consciousness and is source of all healing within the body of all human beings! The power of all healing lies within you, it is not in the hands of the doctors! The doctor is a catalyst that assists you in activating the healing power that already lies within your own being! And whether that power becomes activated or not depends a great deal on the thoughts that are flowing through your mind stream within your mental body and the emotions that those thoughts produce! You're healing process can take off like a rocket or be stifled by the content of the thoughts contained within your own mind stream!

Two people with the same illness go for treatment to the same doctor. He prescribed the same treatment regiment for both people yet one is healed and one is not! Was he a good doctor for one patient and a bad doctor for the other one? I think not! The overall disposition of both patients towards their own healing process was influenced an affected by the thoughts contained in the mind stream of their mental bodies, and the emotions that those thoughts produce! If you can truly grasp the information that I am putting forth here, although it may seem quite simple, the magnitude of its power will generate a quantum leap in your healing process! Your mind is the most powerful tool that you have in your healing process. Please learn how to use it! Your body-consciousness is extremely intelligent, that consciousness rides on the back of the divine energy that is flowing throughout your entire body! However Source-Energy has given you free will and the power to choose what you focus your thoughts on. You have the free will to choose life just as you have the free will to choose death. Where and how you choose to focus your conscious thoughts is an indication of your choice! Activate your healing thoughts coupled with your intention to heal and step into your power. Then there is no disease can stop you!

Chapter 9 – Self Esteem

I would like to speak to you now about the subject of self esteem and how it affected my healing process. My self esteem is the value judgment that I make about myself. The value I assigned to my own existence! This may seem to be quite obvious to you but many times it can be overlooked. I overlooked this aspect of my life for a very long time. What value do I place on my existence? How important is my presence on this earth in my own eyes? What is my value to myself and what is my value to others? Do I honestly feel deserving and worthy to be healed? These questions were of paramount importance to me in my healing process. I needed to be brutally honest in my responses to myself! What was the emotional estimation that I made about my own life? And was I willing to look at myself in the complete nakedness of my own being with total honesty? Yes I was! This was a little painful, never the less it was absolutely necessary to do this if I was going to manifest a true healing in my life.

You may have guessed by now that my self esteem was low because it absolutely was! My stepfather who for much of my childhood I believed was my real father only to find out later that he was not. The fact that this man tried to kill me left me with a sense of being unworthy and not fit to exist on this earth! I say this here because no matter how bad you think your situation is there is always hope and love will find a way if you can find the love within you! The need for self esteem is very important to understand. Like the fish that does not understand the importance of water in its life; I did not understand the importance of self esteem in my life. Understanding this was of paramount importance for me in order to be able to heal. To understand and elevate my consciousness I needed to heal the trauma of my childhood, I needed to grow up! Self esteem provided me with that motivation to do just that, along with my will to live. I am trying to use myself as a vehicle so that you may see how some of what I have been through may relate to you and some of your life experiences. We are all part of the same human race and therefore some things are common to us all. However if you are not willing to see the common denominator between us and how some of these things may apply to you in your life then you are missing the entire purpose of this book!

Please allow the courage that is within you to manifest and take control of your mind so as to guide your thoughts towards the things that will assist you in bringing about the healing you would like to manifest in your life.

Many of you have been struggling for such a long time with so many different factors in your life, and you feel like you just want the pain to stop. But as the great Carl Jung once said; what you resist-persist. Embrace your pain and use it to motivate you to heal! I cannot overstate the value of understanding the importance of self esteem in your healing process and in your life. The tangible things of this life we cannot take with us when we leave this life. However the level of our conscious and spiritual development-that is ours to keep forever! Your heart knows this to be true. You are holding this book in your hands now and I say to you there is absolutely no doubt in my mind or that universal mind that has given life to us all that you are most definitely worthy to heal! If you believe this is not the case you have not yet discovered the Divinity of your own being! You have the power to change that belief and replace it with one that produces a feeling power. Please empower yourself, step into your power and allow the self-healing mechanism of your body to do what it naturally wants to do-heal you! Dare to explore within your own mind and reprogram your beliefs so that you may make any adjustment necessary, needed to build your self esteem to its maximum healing potential! You absolutely have the power to do this! It is my belief that self esteem is essential to exist with or without a body!

I am not a psychiatrist but I believe I have a basic understanding of my own mind and no one will convince me otherwise. I believe that most mothers give their love to their children freely however a father's love is different, it is still most definitely love but it must be earned. Little girls see that daddy loves mommy and kisses her and begin to compete with mommy to earn daddy's affection! Likewise I believe little boys must earn daddy's love also, by getting good grades or hitting that home run, and by doing so they hope to win daddy's approval! However if that approval does not come I believe the self esteem of the child involved will most definitely be affected. We see this behavior manifested in women who are constantly doing things to win the approval of men. We also see this behavior in men who put on this macho attitude to win the approval of women and other men. I believe this behavior is trying to get the unfulfilled needs of childhood met!

In my case I needed to go back in time after the attempt on that little boy's life, and give him the love and comfort that he was crying out for all these years, because that little boy is still very much alive within me to this very day! I needed to validate him and tell him how deserving he truly was and that it was not his fault that his stepfather could not find it in his heart to love him! That no matter what I would always love him; and I would not allow anyone and I mean anyone to ever hurt him again; when I did this-then the healing began for the both us in earnest! I began to believe that we mattered and that going through all that pain made us worthy of all the blessings that life would bestow upon us. I would tell the story of that brave little boy to world and how he helped me heal myself. We would share this story so that many other little girls and boys could be healed also! That through his pain he would bring hopes to others and open them up to the love that is available to them and to us all!

It is my contention that the evaluation of my character is tied to my self esteem. I believe this because after healing my inner child, my sense of self esteem increased follow by a shift in my character. A greater sense of confidence came over me and a feeling of being deserving and worthy of good things that life has to offer began to flow into my life. However I began to notice behavior patterns that I was unaware of before and how these patterns would create a negative self esteem in my life. How I would repress things automatically and place them outside of my conscious awareness to keep my image of myself intact. Other people would tell lies and be dishonest but not me. Other people had big egos but not me. I would quickly see the faults of others but not my own. I would say no one is perfect and I would see the imperfections of others but never look at my own imperfections! In doing this I was creating a sense of false or negative self esteem and the price I paid for doing that was sickness!

To reinforce this false sense of self esteem I would seek outside validation from other people. I created co dependent relationships in order to reinforce my negative self esteem. I did this with other people who also had negative or false self esteem as well, although most of this was being done outside of my awareness. All of this process was totally unconscious at the beginning of my healing journey. I would think to myself if you approve of me I must have value! However other people's approval couldn't hide the fact that I felt valueless within myself. All this was done outside of my awareness until I did the healing work on my inner child! Once I did that healing work my consciousness became flooded with all the things and tactics I would use to create my false sense of self esteem! However once I saw what I was doing now I could begin change it, as I did!

I have always been very competitive and chalked it up to living in a very competitive society however society had nothing to do with it. This competitive nature was tied into my sense of negative self esteem. I was silently in competition with everyone. I need to be better than others to validate myself! I must be better than you in order to feel good about myself. Even if the situation wasn't of a competitive nature I would make it a competition to try and win. By doing so would try to validate my sense of false self esteem! I knew logically that some people are better at doing some things than others. But the need to feed my sense of false self esteem was so great that I had to be first in everything. And if I wasn't I would inflict self punishment upon myself with a vengeance!

I was finally able to release this negative self esteem through forgiveness. I forgave myself but most of all I forgave my stepfather, yes my stepfather, the man who tried to kill me! This was a man who suffered from Post Traumatic Stress after the war. At that time no one ever heard of or even knew what Post Traumatic Stress was. When my step father was sober he was OK but when he drank his demons manifested and no one was safe especially me. He had seen horror like no man should ever have to endure and lived with survivor's guilt all his life! His world was a living hell and he hurt the people closest to him; those of us who loved him the most because he just could not help it. He was only a man, human like the rest of us with all of his flaws. He could not give me what he did not have and he just did not have any love for me; and that's just the way it was!

I had to release him and let go, and accepted the fact that he was just a man–I forgave him. But what did this do for me and why was it healing? I forgave this man after he was already dead so it did nothing to improve our relationship because he was dead. But what it did was improve my relationship with myself! You see I went through a great portion of my life feeling like a victim however the time of my victimization was relatively short, my childhood to be specific. But by continuing to see and place myself in the role of the victim I was giving my power away. I was also attracting other people into my life that would mistreat me so as to validate my feelings of victimization! When I finally saw this process and how it was unfolding in my life it was an AH HA moment of me. There was a tendency to want to inflict self punishment upon myself and that's where the self forgiveness came into play! By forgiving my stepfather I was freeing myself from being a victim. By forgiving myself I was releasing myself from self punishment and in doing so I stepped into my own manhood and I began to heal!

By doing this work my beliefs about this life began to change, because I was seeing things in a different light. It is a true blessing for me to be living in this precious human body. I am a human being with the capacity to think and also feel which means I can appreciate and experience love. This is something I can feel and also share with others. When we are able to forgive ourselves and others we open ourselves up to the power of love that we all truly want to feel. When our pets manifest the love they have for us it brings us joy. When our friends manifest the love they have for us they bring us joy. And when we manifest the love we have in our heart for ourselves we receive the joy that the almighty has placed within our own hearts! This love and this joy have a healing power like no other I have ever witness. It is free because it is truly priceless. It is my belief this love will heal all illness because it healed me and that little boy who resides within me!

Chapter 10 – Self Love

I am a student and I have yet to master the art of self love, I am still learning. And I shall be a student until I exit my body and move on to the next level of life! However I have learned some very important lessons and by mastering these lessons I was granted an extended stay on this earth! If by sharing my understanding with you here now allows you to have any insight into your own journey, then I will have fulfilled the purpose of this book. Please understand that I am not coming from a place of arrogance, nor do I think that I have all the answers! I am merely sharing with you what worked for me coming from the perspective that we are all human beings and as such there are some thing that are universal to all of us. If you are a person who has attain a higher level of growth than the teaching contain in this book please bear with me because I am addressing those who may benefit from what I have learned.

Most everyone is familiar with the term self love it means to love yourself. But how does one go about loving themselves? It is my own personal experience that self-love starts with taking responsibility for yourself. Let's look at what this means starting with the word responsibility, my response ability or the ability to respond to myself. We all have the capability of responding to ourselves, yet many of us do not respond to ourselves at all. Why is this so? In my case I did not respond to my needs because I believed that I did not matter. I inherited this belief from abusive parents. I make this statement here because it is a fact not because I am looking to blame someone for the way I once was. My level of self worth was nonexistent because my step father tried to kill me and my mother for whatever her reasons did nothing to stop him. After this happen I spoke to a reverend and he helped me and I was sent to a reform school until a place open up for me in a home for boys in Chicago. We were the throw away kids! The kids that no one wanted and we knew it, not even our parents wanted us!

My basic foundation at the onset of my life was not a good one. I share this with here not because I am looking for sympathy but to you to let you know that I believe anyone and everyone has the capability to learn how to love themselves, everyone no exceptions! I am a firm believer that what does not kill me will make me stronger and this belief has served me well as it can for you if you allow it. As I grew I began to see the list of priorities in my life and my ranking was very low on that list. My job was more important than me, and my car, even my dog; I just didn't seem to matter in my own eyes! The feeling of love was totally alien to me because I had never experienced it!

I remember being in the hospital in the army on

Christmas day and seeing my roommate's family coming to see him. They were overjoyed to see him and his father wept seeing his son in the hospital bed with Hepatitis on Christmas day. This made me feel a profound sense of loss for a love I never had known! This man was actually crying for his son! I knew then that there was true love in this world. My roommate's father asked if my parents were coming to visit me, I said no they are dead because they were and I left it at that. I saw my roommate's sister and girlfriend in competition to see who was going to sit closest to him on the bed. I felt a hole in my heart that I just could not run away from anymore. But this was my pain so I lay in my bed and kept my mouth shut and silently took the pain. I was not going to spoil my roommate Christmas!

Pain was my constant companion I could trust always that pain would be there for me just like a close friend always by my side. Today I now understand that if I must suffer I will do so for the right reasons, growing pain I accept and embrace otherwise I do not welcome pain into my life anymore. But how does a person turn this attitude of not mattering around? I had to validate myself but how do you validate yourself? I validated myself by seeing and discovering my own value! What are the things I possess that are of value to me and can be of value to others? These were the questions that caused me to search within myself to find answers. I found them because these answers are within all of us. We all have immense value within us we just need to discover it because it is most definitely there!

My first value was that I am willing to give love to others. I found out quite early that it was easier for me to give love than to receive it this was due to lack of self worth. But I was on the road to healing myself and I would change this and if I can do so, so can you! Then I just made the decision that my needs are more important to me than anyone else, if this seems selfish to you so be it! I am not looking for anyone's approval here because I must be able to give love to myself before I can give love to anyone else. Let me expand on what I mean here. Today as I write this I am not at a 100% it is January in New York and quite cold and am a little bit under the weather, I am about at 80% of my normal energy. I am probably like you and I like to give a 100% in all that I do. However today I only have 80% to give but I am writing this anyway; by doing so I am giving all I have to give today which is 80%. So I am giving everything I have. Today 80% is my 100%! I will not beat myself up for the other 20% I do not have to give. By doing so I am giving myself Love!

For me this is one of the most important aspects of self love, being kind to yourself! I had to train myself to do this because I never learned this skill from my parents.

Understand this; parents cannot give you what they do not have! My parents did not have love for me, but that does not mean I will allow myself to go the rest of this life without love! I decided to learn the art of love and I decided to start with myself! Every opportunity life offers me to give love to myself I take advantage of. I want to have good friends so I start by being my own good friend first–this is how I love myself then I can be there for others in friendship!

Many people will blow me off saying this guy isn't saying anything new.

If this is you then you are missing the boat! To know this information mentally is one thing but to know it experientially is something quite profound. Common sense healing is not just about mental knowledge it is about one who knows experientially, deep down to the core of his or her very being! Dare to truly love yourself and experience the power of that love. That in and of itself is truly healing and in that love you are one with the power of the divine!

Giving was my next step. In the beginning I would give to others but for all the wrong reasons. I wanted approval from others. I was seeking from them that which I did not receive from my parents–love! Some people saw this as a weakness within me and used it to get me to do what they wanted – essentially I became a doormat that people would walk all over. All of this in the beginning was outside of my conscious awareness, but as I gradually became aware of this behavior pattern within myself which was a deep seated need for approval; through my self-analysis I decided to put a stop to it!

There was this woman at my job that was very pretty and she would ask me to help her with her work from time to time. As time went on her request increased and it started to get a little out of hand. One Friday she tossed some work at me like I was her employee and told me she must have by 4:30pm and walked away. When 4:30 came around I told her to give me her pay check and she looked at me in amazement and asked me, are you crazy? I told her if I am going to do your job then I want to get paid for it and if I am not, then do your own work; that is what they pay you for! She replied we are not friends anymore! To which I responded we were never friends, a real friend would never ask me to do her job! Some people in the office were watching us including the office manager they broke out in applause. She had told some of our co: workers how much of a jerk she thought I really was because I couldn't say no to her.

I left work on time that day. The following Monday the office manager told me with a smile that little miss pretty one had stayed 2 hours after closing getting that project done! Then Bertha the office manager did something unusual she ask me if she could get me a cup of coffee! I could see that she was extending her hand to me in friendship and said okay. This woman was my senior by 20 years and said to me, I was wondering when you were going to stand up for yourself. I knew you had it in you; never let anyone walk over you James! I am proud of you she said–these words almost brought me to tears. They were words I had always wanted to hear from my parents, although they were coming from a co-worker they were very healing for me! I share this story with you now because courage may manifest in many ways. I was not going to let my need for approval and love to allow me to be a doormat anymore! I stood up for myself and in doing so made a real friend with my office manager. I also began learning self respect and I was learning the lesson of giving love to myself!

Some of you may be thinking what's the big deal you just told a woman to do her job? However those of us who struggle with self esteem issues and have a profound longing for love, know how difficult it can be to say no and stand up for yourself to someone that you find very attractive. It takes guts because every part of you is crying out for the love and approval of that person! This is where the giving comes in you see. Do you have the courage to give yourself the right to say no? You see no matter what I would have done for that pretty woman she had already made up her mind about me, and had told our co; workers she thought I was a jerk! I know this because Bertha the office manager who I became friends with told me so. So it made no difference what I did for this pretty woman, I was always going to be a jerk in her eyes! But by standing up for myself I was giving myself strength and respect. And this was also helping me build a new and positive image of myself, someone worthy of respect and love in my own eyes! No one can ever take that away from me because I have paid the price to own it. And by doing so I was healing myself on multiple levels; this is what common sense healing is all about!

It has been my experience that thinking and self love are interrelated. It has already been stated that your thoughts create your feelings and how you feel affects your health. We as people are train not to think, I mean how to creatively think. Now you may be having a hard time with what I am saying, but hear me out for just a moment. This whole book is based on the premise of common sense! And common sense is just you using the intelligence that you were born with. However we are taught at a very early age to think within the box so to speak, to follow the norm and be like the rest of the other people. However in my case my parents were totally messed up, I did not want to think like them because I didn't want to be like them.

Whenever I would show signs of creative thought I was

attacked in one way or another! As a child I would ask questions like why is there nighttime? The response I would get would be because that's the way it is; stop asking stupid questions! My parents would tell me to do things and I would ask why, not because I was challenging their authority but because I wanted to know the reasons why they wanted me to do what they were asking me to do! The response I got was-because I said so! I was not trying to be rebellious or a brat I was just trying to use my common sense! When I went to school they also just wanted me to "think inside the box" just like everyone else. In school I would ask questions like why is it whenever the Indians win it's a massacre but when the Calvary wins it is a glorious victory! I was told not to disrupt the class. I was beginning to learn at an early age that if my thinking did not conform I would get into trouble. I was suppose to think the way people wanted me to think and that was not think at all! My teachers often would ask me questions like how you could even think of such a thing James; because I have common sense and I would like to use it! I believe my capacity to think is a gift from Source-Energy to me.

Allow me to take this a step further. In high school we read about a Quaker Pastor who would give fire and brimstone sermons that really scared the hell out of the people of his parish. He told them of the fires of hell that awaited them if they didn't change their ways. Then we were given a quiz. A question was asked; why did the pastor give that kind of sermon to the people of church? Everyone answered to scare the people. I answered to get them to repent! When I received my quiz I got a 90%, and I was angry. I ask the teacher, why did you mark that answer wrong? She turns to the class and asks them; class why the pastor give that kind of sermon; they all said in unison to scare the people! This made me even angrier then I stood up from my desk and said you are all wrong! The teacher yelled at me and told to take seat which I did, but I wasn't going to let go of this one because my class mates were laughing at me now! Miss Smith saw I wasn't going to let go of this and said; I will give you a chance to make bigger fool out of yourself James you tell us why the pastor gave that sermon! I said the pastor wanted to control the people of his church and he was using fear to do it! His reasons for wanting to scare them were quite clear to me; he wanted them to modify their behavior and he wanted to get them to repent! This was why he was using fear in the first place. Fear was the means–not the end; the end was to get them to repent! After I spoke the class stopped laughing and I got a 100% on the quiz. I knew that answer because my stepfather used fear to try and control me for most of my young life! Miss Smith never called on me again for the entire year after that!

These are just a few of the many examples we all have about the learning process. We are taught to think within the box and stay within the norm, don't rock the boat if you want to be accepted! Yet all of our greatest men and women had the courage to step outside of the box to become who they truly were as total human beings. My question to you is this; are you willing to step outside of your box? Can you allow yourself to be who you truly are and the hell what others think! Can you get out of your comfort zone and reprogram your thoughts about yourself? Of course you can! But are you willing to do it? You can give yourself love, true love and self respect if you only take that step and use your common sense. If your thinking is flawed and you know it then you do not have to put up with it; be brave because you have the power to change the way you think because you have been blessed with the gift of common sense!

You must be the "Holistic Doctor" of your own consciousness! There is no pill you can take or injection you can get that will do this work for you, at least not that I know of! It is really about looking in the mirror, not the reflective mirror but the mirror of the heart, because you must see who you truly are so you may heal. The power that created us made you incredibly strong and beautiful. Every man and every woman has the power to change but there is a price we must to pay! However there is a price we must pay for remaining the same, the choice is one only you can make. Your feelings will be of great guidance to you in this process. Do the thoughts you have feel empowering, do they give you a sense of strength, if so then you are on the right track. If they are not do not beat yourself up! Just be an observer and watch what is going on with your thoughts.

What you want to do here is just become aware of the habits of your thinking process. Once you have done that you have made a quantum leap in the right direction, you have taken the first step. Our minds are creatures of habit just like us. So discover the habits of the thought process of you mind.

Find out what are the idiosyncrasies that are unique to your own mind. You can allow yourself to have fun with this process like an explorer going into uncharted territories. The approach you have in this process is important. I went into my process with the attitude, I was going to be like Carl Jung and discover new ways to help myself. I was going down the road less traveled, where only the brave dare to tread! I was on the starship enterprise exploring the unchartered territories of my own mind! This can be real fun if you keep the right mindset. Remember to treat yourself with the same love and kindness you would like to receive from others, because you are going to make some mistakes that is part of the learning process. Be kind to yourself for that kindness is another way of you giving love to yourself! Use your common sense and do not be afraid to think outside the box!

This brings us now to awareness, "Self Awareness". I am asking you to discover the thought process of your mind because we have habits and repression is one habit we all have! As a child I was the victim of abuse.

This was a part of my life that I wanted to forget so I repressed that part of my life for many years. However, what I was really doing was disowning my past and that abused child [me!]. I was locking that child away in the basement of my mind! By trying to repress that part of my past, that part of my life [my child] had no voice and could not grieve, and as a result I could not heal! I discovered that I also had a disown youngster, a disown teenager and a disown adult too; by disowning them none of them had a voice to express their pain!

I began to realize that what I was really doing was disowning various aspects of myself; no wonder I was sick! These disowned aspects of me would manifest themselves anyway in very dysfunctional ways, usually hurting the people I cared about the most! I came to the conclusion that I could not run away from me! I needed to heal my child, little junior who they tried to kill; no one else could heal him but me! Then I needed to heal that young boy that never got picked for baseball, then that teenager that the girls would always say no to whenever he ask them for a dance. Finally that adult who decided that it was just too painful to open up and be hurt once again; better off being alone than hurt!

I had to reclaim these parts of myself and give them their voice so that we could finally grieve together! Then and only then could the real healing begin! You see there is a reason I am sharing this information with you here now, and it is not to get sympathy, it is because I would like you to follow the old adage of Socrates *"KNOW THYSELF"*! You see I worked to heal my inner child because I was traumatized as a child. I also understood that I was also traumatized as a young boy, a teenager and an adult. I have healed that child, young boy and that teenager, and I am still working on healing that adult part of me! You see you must know yourself to truly know which aspects of yourself need healing. You see maybe your inner child is okay because your childhood was fine. Perhaps you were traumatized as a young girl or boy due to a separation or a divorce. Or perhaps that part of your life was perfectly okay because it was as teenager when your hormones kicked in, and you had to find your sexual identity and preference for the opposite or same sex when your problems started! Maybe you went through your teenage years just fine, but as a young adult finding your place in society was where you had difficulties.

So when I say to you "**Know Thyself**" by doing so you will attain self knowledge and that self knowledge leads to wisdom! This wisdom is the path to self love! Otherwise yourself love will come from the ego and you will put a smile on your face for others to see while you are dying inside. I speak from personal experience! You see I see good health as a physical, emotional, mental, and spiritual process. Your doctors deal with the physical because that is what they are trained for! When you go to your doctor he gives you something to take care of your physical manifestations of your illness, but the root causes could be mental and emotional and the problem will just reappear in another part of your body later on down the road somewhere else.

It is like when you cut your grass and there is a weed growing, your lawn mower will cut it but it does not get the root of the weed, so the weed will just grow right back! This why I stress that you must be your own 'Holistic Doctor" because you must work in tandem with your doctor, he will do the outer work while you do your inner work. Your doctor needs your help and if you stay on top of your inner work this can also keep you out of the doctor's office! Part of loving yourself is knowing yourself! Are you willing to become aware of the disown parts of your being? Are you willing to embrace your pain and once and for all totally get it out of your system? Are you willing to stop running and face yourself? Do you have the courage to embrace what you have been trying to run away from your whole life? Because if you do you can truly heal yourself! If you will only take that step so that you could see how magnificently beautiful you truly are. No matter how unattractive you think your outer shell may be, your inner beauty is a manifestation of Divine Consciousness! You are truly magnificent and you can change your life! Come over to my side and dare to dream! Dare to fly, dare to walk with the Divine and dare to fall in love with yourself! And let us walk through this life in UNINHIBITED JOY! Because you can do this, you can heal yourself-Yes You Can! Yes You Can!! Yes You Can!!!

Chapter 11 – The Procession of the Equinoxes

This now brings us to the subject of Mother Earth. You may be asking yourself right now, what does the earth have to do with my healing process? I will explain many of you are aware of the predictions of 2012 as stated in Mayan Prophecies. Many people have predicted a global disaster will take place when we arrived at the year 2012. I personally do not believe in any of these predictions, absolutely none of them! I am aware of the Possession of the Equinoxes. Most people are aware that the earth moves through the 12 constellations once every year, Pisces, Aquarius, and Taurus and so on. This movement is like the second hand on your watch. The Possession of the Equinoxes is like the hand on your watch that counts the hours, only each hour consists of 2200 years! We are moving out of the Age of Pisces and into the Age of Aquarius. The actual shift began in earnest in the year 1987 and will complete itself in the year 2012; it is a 25 year shift and we will enter the Age of Aquarius in its entirety in the year 2012. The Mayan astronomers understood this! An astute reader will have recognized that the procession of the astrological signs rotates in a clockwise manner; however the Procession of the Equinoxes rotates in a counter clockwise manner.

Now what does this mean to you and your healing process? The constellation of Pisces is represented by two fishes going in opposite directions. Throughout the past 2200 years we have had a history of the war and war is most definitely conflicting energy. The fish in the constellation of Pisces are going in opposite directions and this represents the conflict.

Also, fish are not conscious that they live in water unless they are removed from it! Please do not misunderstand what I am saying here, I was born under the astrological sign of Pisces so please understand that I am talking about the "The Age of Pisces" which is 2200 years in duration, and not the constellation of Pisces! Now let's look at the "Age of Aquarius". Aquarius is the bearer of water. It is represented by a woman caring a vase of water on her shoulders and is dominated by female energy. Unlike the fish, the Aquarius Woman is very conscious and aware of herself and she brings with her the life-giving substance of water. Unlike the age of Pisces in this age women will not be held in an inferior social status to men! In the Age of Aquarius women will claim their rightful position at the right hand of mankind and let me say here that it's about XXX time! All men presently on the earth have come into the earth through the womb of woman. All of these women have risked death in the process of child birth! I find the fact that they have been forced into a social status unequal to men to be totally ridiculous! However all this is about to change, so guys you better get used to it because like it or not the change is coming!

Mother Earth is undergoing a planetary shift on an energetic level from the Age of Pisces into the energy of Aquarius. The Aquarius Woman brings with her a shift in planetary conscious awareness and an increase of power to the earth, also to all the people on the face of the earth as well. This means you too! Allow me to expand on this point. Let's say you are a child and your mother wins the lottery for 100 million dollars! Your mother now has lots of money now, she can buy you the best clothes, send you to the best schools, and she can give you the best of everything that money can buy.

You will benefit exponentially from all of the money that your mother has come into. I hope you can see where I'm going with this. Our Mother Earth has come into an inheritance of great energy through the coming of the Age of Aquarius. All of her children will benefit from this inheritance of great energy and this includes you! Your illness is nothing more than energy that is out of balance. The energy that you now have access to will blow the socks off of any sickness!

I and others like me are aware of this fact and have discovered the methodology of how to tap into this energy; I am sharing this methodology with you here now. If you are doubtful that is perfectly okay but do not let your doubt stop you from taking action, try this methodology on for size because it works! This is a fantastic time to be alive. We as human beings can now understand how powerful we truly possess; we can do magic! We are co-creators with Source-Energy living on a planet that is coming into an inheritance of great energy. We have an unlimited supply of energy that we can tap into. We only need to open up our eyes and be aware of this fact! It is time for you to step into your power and perform your magic and heal yourself! I am talking to you! Yes you can! Your being on the face of this planet right now is no accident! You are destined for greatness, believe this; if you want to you can heal yourself!

We as human beings living on the earth are energy beings that are constantly vibrating energy, however the earth and everything on the earth is also vibrating with energy. And like energy attracts like energy, because there is a harmonic resonation between the two energy frequencies, your energy frequency and that of Mother Earth. Weather you believe it or not this material you are reading also radiates energy, and its resonation is in harmony with you because you are reading it now! Many of you who are experiencing illness at the present moment may also be going through a purification process! Your body may be attempting to purify itself of toxins so that you may rise to the next level of energy frequency in your evolutionary growth process. This in turn will give you greater energy and make you healthier and stronger! This is not the case with everyone, but there is a good chance that this may be the case in your situation. So please do not see your illness as damnation! Please try to see it as a tool that life is using to teach you more about yourself!

Remember all human beings get sick from time to time, you and I are no exception. However it is also a natural part of the healing process to recover from sickness, and if you are stuck in your illness and are not recovering, this only means you have yet to learn the lesson that your disease is trying to teach you! Once you have learned that lesson the disease will go away, because it no longer serves a purpose being in your body! I hope you can feel what I am saying here; that's right feel what I am saying! Your brain may be reacting to the information that I am now giving you. But if you feel what I am saying your heart knows that this information is true, and will act upon it and this in turn will help you heal! Remember you are the Holistic Doctor of your own consciousness. Your universe, your earth, and your body are all trying to assist you and help you heal! However, you are responsible for enlisting the help of your own consciousness, and no one else can do that for you!

You must remember you are not alone, you have help. Use all of the support systems that you have available to you and also use your family, friends and loved ones if they are there for you. And allow your mind to absorb the teachings that are in this book. There are other books that are on the list of recommended readings that are available to you also, allow your consciousness to focus and be absorbed by them. Remember you have the power to place your consciousness on anything you want. So if you want to heal place your consciousness on the things that will promote healing in your life.

I also say to you here and now that if you are constantly watching TV you are misplacing your focus! You are using television as a means of escape and this does not serve you well. Don't get me wrong I watch TV too from time to time. However I don't live in front of it! Much of the input you receive from TV especially women is constantly telling you directly or subliminally that you are not good enough! Nothing could be further from the truth. If you want to submerge your consciousness into something that will serve you well, I highly recommend that you turn off your TV and turn on your computer. Log on to "Hay House Radio.Com". This is an internet radio station put together by Louise Hay and she has amassed a group of highly developed individuals that are on the cutting edge of conscious development. People like Doctor Wayne Dyer who will take you beyond the traditional concepts of medicine and embraces the total human being! A person like Sylvia Brown who is in my opinion is one of the best psychics on the planet today! You can call the show and actually ask her questions if you like. People like Doreen Virtue who is a highly developed woman who actually channels angelic beings. These are only a few of the many people on this radio show. These people will emerge your consciousness in positivity and will assist you in putting your mind in the yes I can mode of thinking! Louise Hay herself has also had to overcome the life treating illness of breast cancer. These are people that are worth the investment of your free time and can offer insights that can help you on the road to recovery. Through the media of the internet Louise Hay has made these people available to the entire world so take advantage of this asset. You may be asking yourself now how much is this going cost me; not one red cent!

The universe is offering you many opportunities; see the abundance that is available to you and choose wisely. Remember to use your common sense, after all this is what common sense healing is all about!

I have introduced the concept of sickness as teacher, and some of you may still be having a hard time with that. So allow me to expand on the concept here. Anyone who goes though a life-threatening disease and rises above it has learned something meaningful about themselves and life. I speak now for my own personal experience. I understand how precious my human body truly is because it is through this human body that I am allowed to have the gift of life! And when I say to you the gift of life, I truly understand that my life is a gift! I have deep gratitude in my heart for Source-Energy because it has bestowed upon me the gift of this life. This deep sense of appreciation that I have for my life affects the energy that I resonate in my body on a daily basis. This deep sense of gratitude and appreciation in my heart sends my energy out into the universe; it is my way of saying thank you to the Almighty! It is like a child showing its parent exactly how much they appreciate everything that is being done for them.

This appreciation only makes the love between the child and the parent's grow stronger. I am a child of Source-Energy and Source-Energy adores me! This statement does not come from ego or conceit; it comes from the knowledge that I have within me of whose child I truly am. Every breath I take while I am on this earth I consider a blessing. I am grateful for them because every single breath is priceless each and every one of them! I could never have come to this understanding in my life or this appreciation, were not for my Liver Cancer. I once lived my life from a place of great anger feeling like a victim. The feeling I had in my heart was look at what this life is doing to me! As long as I allowed myself to stay in the role of a victim, I could not heal! My Cancer has taught me to step up to the plate and take responsibility for what is happening in my life. Because no matter what if you don't like what is happening in your life you have the power to change it!

What lessons is life trying to teach you through your disease? One of the lessons that life was trying to teach me was the lesson of self love. Love and kindness are traits that we can learn from our parents. However if your parents do not have these traits or you did not learn them from your parents, then life must teach them to you! This was the case with me. I was a hardheaded, difficult student who took 20 years, and almost died in the process of trying to learn the lessons of self love and kindness. Yet I can say to you today that I love being on this earth, I love the children of my Mother Earth, and I love the gift of this life! People; there is a healing power in this love and this love is also inside of you! Do you have the courage to say yes to love and kindness? Do you have the courage to say yes to your life? Are you willing to reprogram unloving bad habits? Are you willing to retrain yourself so you can become the loving human being that you were destined to be? If you answered yes to these questions then you can most definitely heal yourself because you can now learn from your illness. Remember I say to you again you are not alone, Source-Energy will guide you every step of the way. Just keep an open mind and use your common sense!

Chapter 12 – Your Body: The Electromagnetic Field

Scientists have stated that the earth is an electromagnetic field. They have stated that the human body is an electromagnetic field also. What does this mean for the layperson like you and me? What constitutes this electromagnetic field for the earth and what constitutes this electromagnetic field of our body? And what does any of this have to do with the healing process? These were questions I asked myself on my healing journey. I shall share the answers I have discovered with you here now. As you may have recognized by now I am a person that likes to keep things simple. Even the things that seemed to be intrinsically complicated if you break them down to the lowest common denominator they are basically simple. So let's look at the earth and what composes its electromagnetic field. It is pretty much common knowledge that the center of the earth is molten rock. We get a glimpse of its intensity from time to time when we see the eruptions of a volcano. The center of the earth's core along with the heat it produces constitutes the electrical factor of the earth's electromagnetic field. The major portions of the surfaces of the earth are covered with water and this water constitutes the magnetic factor of the earth's electromagnetic field.

This is also indicative by the fact that water is an

excellent conductor of electricity, water being the magnetic factor, feminine in its energy, and the heat in the earth's core constitutes the electrical factor being masculine in its energy. Although these energies are opposite in their nature they coexist together in perfect harmony. This electromagnetic field constitutes the beautiful blue planet we live on. Our physical bodies are also a reflection of the electromagnetic field of our Mother Earth.

It is common knowledge that our bodies are composed mostly of water.

Scientist says that over 90% of our body is made of water. This water constitutes the magnetic factor of our bodies, and is feminine its energy just like the feminine aspect of our Mother Earth! It is also of common knowledge that our brain discharges electrical impulses. These electrical impulses that are discharged from the brain constitute the electrical factor of our body's electromagnetic field, and this energy is masculine in its nature just like the masculine aspect of our Mother Earth! I hope you can see how our physical bodies are a reflection of the body of the Earth Mother that we live on, not on a physical level but on an energetic one! Now what does this mean and how does this influence the healing process? The masculine and feminine energies of the earth coexist in perfect harmony and will automatically readjust themselves as an imbalance occurs.

The human body has the capacity to do the same thing! What are the representations of this masculine and feminine energy within our human bodies? It is my experience that the masculine aspect of my body is the core of my thoughts and the feminine aspect is the core of my emotions. My brain through my thoughts is constantly discharging electrical impulses throughout my body. These thoughts are affecting and influencing my emotions and how I feel.

These emotions and feelings cause me to take actions. They are the masculine and feminine factors of my body and they work in tandem! Just as the masculine and feminine energies of our Mother Earth work in tandem.

If I am to maintain a state of good health, I must maintain the balance of my masculine and feminine energies within my own body. I hope you can see why I say that the body in my opinion is a mirror of our Earth Mother.

The energies of the human body are kept in balance by the hormones of testosterone and estrogen. Estrogen is the aspect of feminine energy, testosterone the masculine. Every man has a feminine quality within him because he has the hormone estrogen and every woman a masculine quality within her because she has the hormone testosterone! The endocrine system is responsible for the regulation of these hormones within the human body. For a woman to be healthy, she has to have the proper balance of testosterone and estrogen. And for a man he must have the proper balance of estrogen and testosterone. If an imbalance occurs that person will become sick and if the imbalance is severe and left untreated, then that person may have a stroke!

This brings me to my next subject, the subject of men bashing and women bashing! You may be asking yourself now, what on earth does this subject have to do with the healing process? I will explain. I have seen many instances where women come together for a girl's night and they love to indulge in one of their favorite past time, men bashing. Men actively participate in this pastime as well! This past time does not serve you well at all! You may be asking yourself why, what is the harm in this? I enjoy it, it is fun. It makes us laugh, and after all we are different aren't we? Yes we are different and this may seem like a harmless activity on an emotional level.

However on an energetic level its long term effects can be very devastating to your body! As I stated earlier the body maintains health and proper balance through the hormones of testosterone and estrogen. It is the responsibility of the subconscious mind to maintain hormonal balance along with your endocrine system. Your subconscious mind takes orders from your conscious mind. When you indulge in this activity of bashing as innocent as it may seem, you are unconsciously sending signals to your subconscious mind.

Remember your thoughts create your emotions and your emotions affect your body! If you are with a group of women and you are indulging in the activity of men bashing you are unconsciously sending a signal to your subconscious mind! And remember your subconscious mind thinks in pictures. So stop to think about the pictures that you are sending the subconscious mind!

It is my contention that your subconscious mind will see this as a signal to produce less testosterone, even though that is exactly what you do not want. It is also my contention that this in turn can make you sick or even contribute to causing a stroke! I believe this is also true for men as well!

Let's just say for the sake of making a point that your heart receives blood from the left side and pumps out blood from the right side of your body. The left side of your body, the receiving side would be the feminine side and the right the masculine. You would not take a hammer in your left hand and beat your right hand would you? This is exactly what you are doing when you indulge in the activity of men or women bashing! Please do not misunderstand what I am trying to say here. As men and women sometimes we do need to blow off steam and that is perfectly OK! If you have an argument with your boy friend or girl friend, or your husband or wife, it is perfectly normal to seek the companionship of your friends to blow off a little steam. As a matter of fact, if this situation occurs it is healthy to so!

However once you blow off your steam, STOP! Please don't go on a rampage for hours and hours, for the only one you are hurting by doing this is yourself. Your words have power sometimes even beyond your own recognition! So after you have blown off your steam chill out! Remember just use your common sense and you can't go wrong, you will know when you have blown off your steam and when you are crossing the line into excess!

You see by indulging in the activity of bashing what you are really doing is, if you are a woman you are not appreciating the masculine qualities within you! And you are projecting that dislike outward on to your partner so you don't have to see or accept these masculine qualities within yourself! And if you are a man you are also doing likewise! By doing this what you are really doing is performing self rejection! And as I already stated by doing this on a long term basis you are disrupting the hormonal balance within your own body and this can manifest disease! Remember our Mother Earth has both of these energies and they coexist in perfect harmony that is how she stays healthy. We can maintain a healthy body by following her example! Appreciate the totality of your being, both in its masculine and feminine aspects. You have the power of God within you, your masculine energies represents that power! You have the power of the Goddess within you, and your feminine energies represent that power also! By bashing you are placing these energies in conflict with one another, and if left alone they would find a way to work in harmony. By indulging in bashing you put yourself in conflict with the essence of your true nature. Appreciate and accept the wholeness of your total being both in its masculine and feminine aspects! By doing so you will be accepting yourself and taking a step into real self love which in turn will help you heal! This will benefit you mentally, emotionally, and physically. It will also help you stay in and maintain a state of good health. I speak from my own experience.

I once knew a gay woman who totally hated men and she had a heart condition that caused her to require open heart surgery which she did in fact have. She was placed on a heart transplant list to receive a transplant. I spoke with her before she went into the hospital and gave her a reading. The information was coming in from her mother who had cross over to the next level of life. She was concern for her daughter and told me to tell her to have her endocrine system checked. However as I stated this woman hated men and because the information was coming from me, a man she blew me off in a very hostile manner, even though I was offering this information to her absolutely free. She went into the hospital and ten days later she had a severe stroke!

Yet none of this had to happen. I'm not saying that her heart condition would have vanished, however she did not have to go through the pain of the stroke, her mother was trying to warn her and did so through me.

However she couldn't accept the information because it came from a man! I am a man writing this material, and I do not claim to be an expert on the subject of women, however I know one thing and that is I love women!!!

And I could not envision my world without them. Yet women are just as much a mystery to me as they are to the next guy, and I wouldn't want it any other way! I find it to be a mystery that adds the spice to life! And each and every woman is completely unique as is each and every man! I am glad we are different and as they say in France Viva La Difference!

I hope I have made my point clear because although it is a simple one it is in fact very important. Self love and acceptance are of paramount importance in our healing process. And the acceptance I am talking about is the acceptance of our total being; both masculine and feminine! Let me take this a step further. Let say you are a woman and I ask you to describe your fantasy man, aside from being rich and handsome you would probably say that you would want him to be warm, kind, sensitive, caring and loving.

These I would consider to be feminine qualities. If you

ask me to describe my fantasy woman aside from being beautiful I would say I want her to be outgoing, a go getter, she sees what she wants and goes after it, she speaks her mind and stands up for herself. These I would consider masculine qualities. So what are we really saying? You are saying you want a man that is in harmony with his feminine side! I would be saying I want a woman who is in harmony with her masculine side! And we both would be saying we want a total human being! So let us embrace our opposite sides and become the total human beings that we are meant to be, by doing so we can experience greater love and health in our lives. We can expedite the healing process and become whole, and learn the lessons that we came into the earth plane to learn. Let us use our common sense and forgive ourselves for our imperfections, and activate our common sense healing so that we may heal!

Chapter 13 – Your Telephone to Source Energy

Today we live in the age of the cell phones. Nearly everyone has a cell phone. They are useful and quite practical and they definitely come in handy especially in an emergency. It is kind of hard to think of life today without them because they keep us connected to our family, friends, love ones, and our work place. It would be difficult to stay connected to them without a cell phone, let's face it cell phones help us stay connected. We are all connected to Source-Energy but somehow some of us feel we have lost our cell phone connection to our internal source! Some of us feel like we are disconnected from Source-Energy and that we don't have that cell phone to make that call so we that can reconnect! However this is just not true even though we believe the opposite is the case.

Let's picture a mother whose child is going on their first trip away from home. The mother being a parent concern for the well being of her child gives that child a cell phone and says to her child if you have any problems, or need to speak with me for any reason whatsoever don't hesitate to call me! When we left our true home to come into these flesh garments, and incarnated as human beings to go to earth school, our Divine Mother gave us all a cell phone! However many of us have forgotten that we even have that internal cell phone connection to our Divine Mother, which is our "Source Energy". This does not mean that we do not have it, because it is standard equipment for all human beings and this includes you! You may be asking yourself now what is this guy talking about? If you have a serious illness you probably have ask yourself as I did why is this happening to me? You have probably search within yourself for answers and come up short. When I searched within my mind for answers and came up empty, I still needed answers only I needed to look to a source that was higher than my own mind to find them. I did not have the answers and the doctors did not have the answers either. That's when my cell phone connection became a hot item. I knew that the power that gave me life could also give me the answers I needed to help me heal! But I had forgotten how to contact my Divine Mother. I struggled with this situation for quite some time and when I finally found the answer I felt like such an idiot because it was sitting right there before me the whole time! To contact my Divine Mother all I needed to do was to place my hands together over the center of my chest or "the heart chakra" for those of you who are familiar with this terminology, with the intention of talking to her; it is that simple! We recognized this as the prayer posture; it is a universal posture for all mankind. If you go to China and see someone performing this posture you know what it means, if you go to Australia and see this posture you know what it means, anywhere in the world you go it means the same thing for all human beings! It makes no difference what your religious denomination is, weather you are a Christian or a Moslem, of the Jewish faith, a Hindu or Buddhist. You are still a child of the Divine Mother and this posture connects you to her! Children instinctively know this posture as well. Like I said it is standard equipment for all human beings. It may seem like I am stating the obvious here because I am, however sometimes we tend to overlook the obvious, I know I did.

There is also a very important factor to remember here and that is your intention! If you are just going through the motions then this means nothing, but if your intention and desire is to consciously communicate with your Divine Mother which is that Source-Energy then that call goes through every single time; no exceptions! Many people feel they already know this, yet to know this mentally is one thing-but to know this experientially is something completely different; it is that Ah Ha!!! The moment when the light bulb goes on and you totally get it. If you just use your common sense here you can't go wrong. And you will understand that little difference that makes the big difference! Call home your Mother is concern about you!

Now if you are wondering why you have developed this sickness and perhaps even what it is that your sickness is trying to teach you, you can now use your cell phone to call Source-Energy and ask your questions. Once you put in your request for answers then sit and meditate and wait for your response. If you are a person with no meditative experience do not despair! So what if you don't know how to meditate! You know how to sit in a chair with your back comfortable straight and allow yourself to relax don't you?

Then do that and just relax your breathing and you will be just fine! Eventually you will notice that the volume of your thoughts becomes softer. The volume of those thoughts will lower itself from 10 to about maybe 3 or 4.

When this happens just be quiet and just listen. Your answers will come; it would be painful for your Divine Mother not to come to you and comfort you-her child! However let go of your concepts of how this is going to happen because your answers can come in many ways, so keep an open mind. Above all be patient if you don't get your answers the very first time that's okay. Sometimes the phone may have to ring a few times before it gets picked up! Just be clear on your intention and expect your answer to come; your expectation is the magical ingredient, your call will be answered! Now you must be brave, I say this to you because you may not like the answers you get. The answer I got when I put in my request to what was the lesson my illness was trying to teach me was self love! My ego reacted violently to this answer and my anger just made me sicker! Common sense healing is simple but I didn't say that it was easy, sometimes it can be but sometimes the lessons that we need to be learned can be very hard. However the harder the lesson the greater the breakthrough! Please remember this because it will serve you well on your journey to recovery. Remember this is a process of self discovery and the person you need to discover and fall in love with is you! When you can do this you are on the road to rapid recovery. If you think this statement does not apply to you, let me ask you just one question; do you ever beat yourself up? My answer to this question was a definite yes because I didn't feel worthy, and I was trying to be perfect so I could become worthy in my own eyes! Let me say to you here and now that if I was in fact perfect there would be no need for me to be here on the earth plane because there would be nothing here for me to learn. Remember this is earth school and we come here to learn! So be patient and wait for your answers and when they manifest be open to them! If they are painful embrace the pain for it is a good pain; it's a growing pain and by embracing it you will step into your power and you will heal! You can actually make this discovery process fun; putting together the puzzle of your life is exciting. When you actually start to see an improvement in your health you know that you are mastering the process. Then you will understand what I have been saying about stepping into your

171

power and oh what rush it is to feel the power of your divinity! Once you have learned this process it is yours, you have paid the price to master it and no one can ever take it away from you!

I was treating my friend Karen she was complaining about having some chest pains and came over for a session. She and I go back a long way and I care about her a great deal. Normally her situation is very easy to treat, and with one session, two at most would be all it takes to restore her energy back into harmony and into balance. However she was not responding and I was beginning to get a little worried. Karen is also a quite competent healer in her own right and I knew something was going on with her but I just couldn't put my finger on it. After a session a person's energy is usually much stronger but this was not the case with Karen. I knew this was cause for concern, so I decided to talk to her about it. So when the session was over I ask her Karen, why do you think you are still having these chest pains? She answered I don't know with a tone of hostility! Karen is a woman with a strong personality and can be very intimidating and she uses this to keep people at a distance sometimes. I care about her and I saw right through what she was doing. Karen you know something is going on with you and so do I, I said. You can slap my face if you must but I am not going to back off until we both know what's going on with you. She gave me that stare that women can give you to intimidate the hell out of you, but this was a friend of mind and I was not going to back off! Again she answered with hostility I don't know! I decided to change my approach. Karen you are a highly competent healer and you know there is a reason why these chest pains are not going away. If it was just an energy imbalance it would have corrected itself by now especially with these sessions. What do think it might be? Her demeanor softens a bit but again she replied I don't know.

Karen you are in your head I said, don't think for the answer feel for it! Your brain is repressing this answer because it is something painful that it doesn't want you to deal with. You are a healer and you know that your body knows the answer because you body has intelligence and consciousness! Let your body give you the answer not your brain! She became very quiet and then she began to tremble. I sat quietly with my friend, and then she spoke as tears began to form in her eyes. She said, I think Johnny is cheating on me!

Johnny has been seeing another woman and I have seen them together. Then she went on to describe this woman and I knew who she was. This woman was young and very attractive and she is in the catering business. I knew Johnny was planning a surprise party for Karen for their tenth anniversary because I was invited to it. My dilemma now was should I spoil the surprise or let my friend suffer. I was not going to let Karen suffer like this; surprise party be dammed! So I spilled the beans and told her what was going on. A sense of relief came over her and we laughed together.

I am sharing this story with you here to make the point about body consciousness! Karen's mind was repressing what she was not ready to deal with, however her body knew exactly what was causing her pain! When I use the term your Emotional Body I want you to understand that your emotions are an aspect of your subconscious mind and that your emotions or your [emotional body] takes orders from your conscious mind, that is your [mental body]! Karen's conscious mind perceived a betrayal even though Johnny was not betraying her! Her conscious mind; or [mental body] decided not to acknowledge this situation because the thought of it was too painful for her to bear! However her [emotional body] or subconscious mind knew exactly what was hurting her. Even though she did a pretty good job of repressing that thought of betrayal, the results of that repression caused her to have chest pains! It is no coincidence that the pains manifested in her chest because that is where the heart is located and the thought of Johnny betraying her was breaking her heart! This is just common sense!

Your body knows the truth because the ultimate truth is who you are and your body resonates with that ultimate truth! Use your cell phone to contact "Source Energy", but always remember all the answers are within you, your body knows! That ultimate intelligence that is Source-Energy knows exactly what you are capable of handling. Timing in healing is of the utmost importance. Certain medications need to be taken at a certain time for maximum effect. Certain things need to be understood at a certain time for the maximum healing benefit. And Source-Energy always knows when it is the perfect time for you. Your "Source" will never let you down, ever! Trust your "Source", trust your body and trust your common sense. This is how you use common sense healing!

Chapter 14 – Seeing in Believing

Now I would like to talk to you about the creative mind and its power to visualize. Whenever I want to manifest something from thought into physical manifestation, it always helps me when I have a clear image of what I want to manifest in my mind. This is something I do consciously and by doing this consciously I am also enlisting the help of my subconscious mind. Remember, as it has already been stated that your subconscious mind thinks in pictures! The clearer the picture the easier it is to bring that picture into manifestation. I am assuming that you are reading this book because you want a healthier body. So see yourself already in possession of the healthy body you desire. If your body was 100% healthy right now what would you do? How would you behave? Where would you go? Let me explain the point I'm trying to make by using an analogy. When I was afflicted with my Liver Cancer the one thing I wanted to do most was walked barefoot on the beach. However walking barefoot in the sand on the beach can make a healthy person tired, for someone with liver disease like myself that was totally out of the question. The fatigue would have been too great for my body to endure! However this was something that really loved doing when my body was healthy. So I would take the time to sit down and relax my mind and see myself doing just that, walking on the beach. I would feel the warm sand underneath my feet and smell the salt water of the ocean. I would feel the sunshine gently caressing my face and the ocean mist gently blowing on my body. And I would feel the joy and invigorating feeling of how it felt to be healthy once again walking on the beach! My body would be radiating happy energy, and I would have a big smile all over my face.

My subconscious mind would see these images that I was sending to it and would act upon those images, because this was what I truly wanted. Remember that your subconscious mind thinks in pictures and you have the power to send to your subconscious mind the pictures of what you want!

Allow me to use another example here. Let's say there is a child, and that child wants a bicycle for Christmas. The child approaches the parents and says I know what I want Santa to bring me for Christmas. The parents reply what sweetheart? The child answers I want Santa to bring me a bicycle. Then the child goes on to describe in vivid detail exactly the kind of bicycle that they want. As the child describes this bicycle the parents can see the excitement in the child's face, there is a joy in the child eyes that makes their parents smile. That mother and father now understands what will make their child truly happy and now know exactly what to get their child for Christmas. The child has communicated quite clearly exactly what it wants. The parents have received this communication loud and clear. And they now know exactly what to get their child for Christmas; it would be painful for them not to have a bicycle under the Christmas tree for their child on Christmas day! There is no doubt in the child's mind that Santa is going to deliver on their request. The child expects with 100% certainty that on Christmas day that bicycle will be there!

It is this expectation of certainty that pulls at the parents heart strings. The mother and father will not disappoint their child! You are the child and the subconscious mind is the parent in this case! Just as your subconscious mind is trying to do everything in its power to keep you alive and healthy, it will do everything in its power to keep you happy also. However it is of Paramount importance that you be totally clear on what it is that you want! And that your expectation should be exactly like that child, a 100% certainty that it will manifest. Do not wish for it; do not hope for it, you must expect it with a 100% certainty!

The term visualization can be intimidating for some people, if you are one of those people then do not think of the term visualization. Substitute the term visualization with imagination or fantasizing. Remember to keep this simple and just use your common sense! Sometimes the initial knee-jerk response that most people have is that I can't do this. Yes you can! Everyone knows how to fantasize and dream. This includes you also, so empower yourself, and dare to dream of the healthy body that you desire. You may be a person who falls into the category of one who believes that nothing works for me. This only means that you have some unconscious habits that cause you to self sabotage! You may be thinking to yourself now, these habits are unconscious; I don't even know that I am doing them, and you would be right! However just because these habits are unconscious now, that does not mean that you cannot bring them to into your conscious awareness! Place yourself in a relaxed state by finding a quite place to sit and relax. Then ask yourself how can I bring myself sabotaging habits into my conscious awareness? When you ask yourself this question, how can I see myself sabotaging habits, especially when you do it from a relax state, you will be engaging the help of your subconscious mind. If you keep asking yourself this question consistently from a relaxed state, the subconscious mind we bring the answers into your awareness for you. I speak from personal experience, and if you do this technique consistently you will be able to speak from your personal experience also! This technique works for most people however if you are one of those persons that cannot employ this technique successfully, then I suggest that you pray. Because prayer is also another way in which you can engage the subconscious mind. And you definitely know how to pray. Ask Source-Energy to reveal to you the techniques that you are using that causes you to self sabotage in your life. Ask and it is given each and every single time!

The process of visualization, of imagining or fantasizing will transmit the pictures of what you want to your subconscious mind. When these pictures become crystal clear your subconscious mind will act upon them. The old adage; "Seeing is Believing" truly applies here. Because when you're subconscious mind has a clear picture it acts upon it because that that is what you want. For your subconscious mind -"Seeing is Believing"! If you are in need of more guidance on this subject please read "The Power of Your Subconscious Mind" by Joseph Murphy. It is written in a clear and simple manner so even a 10 year child can understand it, it is a masterpiece; I highly recommend it!

Chapter 15 – Meditation

At this point I would like to talk to you about the subject of meditation. Many of you may already be familiar with meditation. However for those of you are not, let me demystify it for you! There are many different forms of meditation. The meditation I would like to introduce to you here is a very simple and basic one. The only requirement that is necessary is that you are alive, because if you are alive then you are breathing, and that is all you need to do this meditation! The things that tend to be most powerful and effective in our lives are usually the most simple. And this is also the case with this meditation. This meditation is called "Baby Breathing" and it is something that you already know how to do. The only thing I will do is show you how to get back in touch with it. The first thing you need to do is find a comfortable place to sit and relax. You can sit on the floor on a cushion with your legs crossed if you find this position comfortable for you. Or you may sit in a comfortable chair if you prefer. The only two basic requirements are that you keep your back as straight as is comfortably possible, and above all that you relax. Then as you sit I would like you to bring your attention to your breathing, and allow it to become as effortless as the breathing of the newborn child! If you have ever observed a new born child laying in its crib its breathing is totally effortless. There is absolutely no thought process happening there. Source-Energy is just breathing that child. You are also a child of Source-Energy and Source-Energy is also sustaining and breathing you!

If I had to remember to breathe I would be dead, because my nature as a human being is forgetful! Yet every night when I go to sleep Source-Energy always remembers to keep me breathing and gives me the breath of life!

This requires absolutely no effort on my part. There is a divine rhythm happening just like a mother sitting in a rocking chair holding her child who she gently rocks back and forth. So just focus on that rhythm of the breath and allow that divine mother that is your Source-Energy to rock you! Just sit on your comfortable cushion or chair and bring your attention to your breathing, and then allow it to relax and become as soft and effortless as the breathing of a newborn child. You will be amaze at how peaceful and comforting this experience can be. You will be coming home to who you truly are merely by relaxing into that divine breath that is sustaining you.

This in and of itself is a truly healing experience.

Remember allow your breathing to be as soft and as effortless newborn child. If you find this to be difficult I highly recommend that you go to a hospital and watch a newborn child sleeping, see how relax and peaceful it truly is. This is the same peaceful relaxation that Source-Energy wants to bestow upon you. It is your birth right because you are a human being; you are a child of the "Divine"! There is no time factor here you may sit as long as you like. If your thoughts tend to come up do not step into them and don't try to force them to go away, just allow them to be there! And bring your attention back to your breathing and allow it to be as soft and effortless as a newborn child, and eventually your thoughts will subside.

I cannot overstate the power of this simple yet profound meditation. It is "Source Energy's" gift to you, a way for you to get out of your thoughts and be with the essence of who you truly are; but most importantly it will also help you heal! However if it does not click for you the very first time you try it-don't give up! Just try it again and eventually you will get the hang of it, and not only will you get it-you will master it. So stay with this process because you are well worth it! I would like you to be aware of each time you inhale because when you inhale you are taking in the breath of life from Source-Energy and with every exhale you are giving that breath of life right back. There is a gentle rhythm taking place here and that rhythm is the rhythm of life! It is just like a mother sitting in a rocking chair rocking her child. Allow yourself to feel and experience this rhythm; for it is the breath of life that can heal all sickness! The beauty of this meditation is that if it done properly it is truly effortless, all that is required of you is that you focus and relax your breathing and allow it to become as soft and effortless as a new born child that is all. There is no doubt in my mind that you can do this because you are breathing. That is really all it takes, just that and a little common sense, after all this is common sense healing! Allow yourself to be the child that you truly are and just relax, it really is just that simple!

I highly recommend that if you are new to meditation that you go through this process for 21 consecutive days, that way you will develop the habit of meditating on a consistent basis. As you do this you will begin to experience the many benefits that this process can produce. It would benefit you to practice in the morning and at night, however if this isn't possible then pick a time that is good for you and practice at that time on a daily basis. Do not make this into hard work because it does not have to be work at all. Allow this to be a labor of love! Let me also state here that resistance will come up! And it is perfectly normal. Your reactive mind will resist the fact that you are attempting to practice a discipline, because your reactive mind wants to be in control of you! Do not listen to all the objections that your reactive mind will throw in your face, telling why it is just not possible for you do to this for 21 days. You have been listening to your reactive mind a lot and it is pretty much in the driver's seat.

It will resist you trying to regain control of your life. However rest assured that one of the contributing factors to your disease is that you have allowed your reactive mind to be in charge!

Take control of your life because your life depends on it! When I first went through this 21 day process my reactive mind was all over me, just like a spoiled brat wanting to have its way. But I am the one who calls the shots in my life, not my reactive mind! I did something that was very helpful for me that I wish to share with you here. I broke this 21 day process down into three weeks. After I finished the first week I considered that as completing elementary school and I took myself out to dinner to celebrate. When I finished the second week I considered that graduating high school and treated myself to a Japanese dinner. And when I finished the finale week I consider that finishing healing college. I had used the power of my will to create a productive habit that was going to help me heal myself. And once again I treated myself to a wonderful Italian meal! This was just another way I chose of giving myself appreciation and love.

Find ways to validate yourself and give yourself love every chance you get on your healing journey! It is an investment you are making in yourself and the dividends are quite beneficial. You may be asking yourself what kind of dividends he is talking about. If your reactive mind hits you with a lot of thoughts, the volume of these thoughts may be very strong, let's say they are at 10 on the volume meter. Meditation can lower that volume to 3, or 4, thereby allowing you to perceive the voice of you inner guidance system, and the guidance that you can receive from your inner guidance system can assist you in healing your body! You have the Knowledge of all Knowledge's vibrating within you. Meditation can assist you in tapping into the tranquility of that Knowledge! And that can bring you inner peace, which in turn will help you heal! I ask you here and now do you have the courage to make this simple 21-day investment in yourself? Are you truly ready to say yes to your life and yes to good health? Are you willing to overcome the self limiting beliefs and concepts you have, by looking them right in the eyes and saying to yourself, I will accept these self imposed chains no longer? I deserve to be healthy, happy and loved! I will start right now, right here where I am at this very moment! If you would like to explore this meditation on a deeper level I highly recommend you go to www.findingout.org which is the website of Prem Rawat who can instruct you in the techniques of Knowledge, he is the one who has taught me! There is also a very good audio meditation called Holosync. If you have seen the hit DVD *The Secret* you saw Bill Harris, who has developed an audio technology that can expedite your development exponentially. I have been using it for about two years now and I endorse it. Bill Harris will send you a free introductory CD. All you pay is the shipping. If you are interested in finding out more, go to www.centerpointe.com . I say to you again that you are not alone; whatever assistance I can offer I am more than willing to do so, just go to my website at www.commonsensehealing.net and E-mail me, whatever assistance I can offer to encourage you on your healing journey I will. Remember encouraging words have the power to help you heal, so don't be afraid to say them to yourself!

This brings us to our next topic and that is support. You may have family and friends that support and encourage you and that is a good thing. However if they are not supportive or want to put you down or make fun of you because you are involved in things that they do not understand, do not waste your time sharing with them these aspects of your healing process. I also recommend that you not try to convince them or change their minds.

Allow them to think whatever they think about your process. Just remain true to the path of self-healing that you have chosen. You must keep all toxic thoughts and emotions at bay and if your family and friends are contributing factors in bringing toxic thoughts and emotions to you, it would behoove you to keep them at bay also. It is quite possible that they may be doing this totally unintentionally, but if they are do not allow yourself to receive input from them, only you can make the judgment call here! Listen to your heart and do what feels right to you. Remember you must be your own best friend! No matter what you will always have the support of "Source Energy", so, no matter how alone you may believe you are Source-Energy is always available to you, because you are a child of that Divine Source-Energy and you are not alone! Please remember this; you can always talk to "Source Energy," always! This will serve you well in times of doubt; you are not alone, there is much love here for you!

Chapter 16 – Stepping into Adulthood

We come to a subject now that is one that many people want to bypass, over look or just not deal with altogether. And that is stepping into adulthood. It has been my experience that one does not step into adulthood merely with the passing of time. Many of us know of people who are in adult bodies but have yet to grow up! There was once a time in my life when I was one of those people so I speak to you from a personal experience!

Stepping into manhood and womanhood was once a rite of passage in earlier cultures. However today in our so called modern society this is usually not the case. Young men may go into the military and young women can get married or pregnant and in doing so believe that now I am a mature young man or women. However if we take the time to truly examine this we find that this is usually not the case. It is my contention and the premise of common sense healing that stepping into manhood and womanhood is an ever unfolding journey; one does not arrive at this destination merely by the passing of time. It is something that requires courage because we must be willing to face ourselves and the naked truths of who we think are. You may be wondering why I have used the term – [who we think we are]. It is not a misprint. Many of us are running from ourselves trying to hide from others the things we believe are not acceptable about ourselves. By doing so we participate in the process of self rejection! We only do this because we do not see the beauty of the nature of who we truly are. By doing so the process of self discovery which is supposed to unfold for us does not, and we do not fulfill one the purposes of coming into this life–"Know Thyself"!

We all have certain beliefs; I know I did–the beliefs of being unworthy of love, happiness and success. These beliefs were very painful for me to look at and so my conscious mind repressed them out of my awareness into my subconscious mind for years! To step into my manhood I had to become conscious of these beliefs and have the courage to face them in order to become the man Source-Energy wanted me to become. And if I told you that this process was easy I would not be telling the truth because I had to overcome my fears. To do so first I had to admit I had fears in the first place, and then I had to face them to overcome them! However if I did not go through this process you would not be reading this book today. It is your divine inheritance to step into your manhood and womanhood; by doing so you will realize that you are one with the Divine. This is how we truly heal ourselves by discovering our true magnificence. This is why I came into earth school in the first place–to go through this process!

And yes pain is part of the process by which we learn and grow that's just the way it is, this was something I had to learn to accept! However by doing so I was able to finally step into my manhood and now I have self knowledge that no one can ever take away from me!

I came into this life with nothing but I do not leave empty handed. This is not a statement of arrogance or of ego but of self love, I have earn the right to say this; I am my father's son not my physical father-my Divine Father! I am my mother's child not my physical mother-my Divine Mother! I say to you now step over to my side and pay the price to know who you truly are because you are most definitely worth the effort and you do have the courage within to discover the magnificent of the beautiful being that you truly are!

Allow me to tell you about two women I know, one who is not ready to step into her womanhood yet and one who has done so a long time ago. I will tell you of Lynn who isn't ready yet to take that step to becoming all she is destined to be just yet. I have no doubt that she will get there in her own time. She is just overcome by fear-but her fear will pass in time! Lynn came to me recommended by someone I know. She was having problems and believed that she frightens people away from her and that there something was terribly wrong with her. Although she believed this to be true I assure you that this was not the case. However this is what she believed and because she believed this she manifested situations in her life that would validate this belief! She went to see an acupuncturist whom she had an attraction to. During the session she had an energy release of a blockage she had in her heart center. She claimed that the response to the release had frightened her acupuncturist because this was a first time experience for him. And that her response freaked him out! She used this to reinforce the belief that she frightens people and no one understands her.

This no one understands me belief I call the martyr syndrome. She uses this belief to keep herself in victim mode as well. As stated earlier when a person is in victim mode they take no responsibility for what they create in their life, which is exactly what she was doing! I pointed this out to her on several occasions but she defended her position with a vengeance and I was accused of not understanding her and being insensitive, this by the way is a typical response. Most of the times when she called, it was an emotional emergency that required my immediate attention-this was how she created the drama in her life! Her spirit guide communicated with me a suggested I do a healing process with her and interpret her dreams because she would be giving her messages through the dream state. This I did and she received a powerful communication through the dream state. When I interpreted her dream she was very moved by it, so much so that it brought her to tears. She was very near to having her first breakthrough and was about to make some serious forward momentum. Then a situation came up for her and she needed to make a choice, however she wanted me to tell her what to do. This I would not do because by doing so I would have created a codependent relationship between her and me. I was not willing to do that because I wanted to empower her to be able to receive guidance from within herself!

My advice to her was to relax and reflect and her answer would come. And even if she made a mistake she could only learn from it! Then she came at me with the no one understands me stuff looking for sympathy and pity. She finally got that I was not going to support her if this was the path she chose. I would not be a part of her creating a codependent relationship with me, no matter how much she paid me!

The next day we spoke and she discontinued her healing process because "I didn't understand her"! Allow me to clarify a point here. There are some people who are very highly developed on a spiritual level and many of us have difficulty understanding them and their motivation. Their level of consciousness is beyond our scope of comprehension! However these individuals because of their level of development are very compassionate and when we don't understand them their response is one of love and compassion not anger! Lynn response was anger on the borderline of rage.

This is indicative of a person who does not understand their self. And they project blame on to others when they do not receive what they want from them! I held up a mirror and Lynn didn't like what she saw, failing to realize that I was there for her if she was willing to the work needed to change and grow. She was so close to a real breakthrough but she wasn't quite ready to pay the price. It saddens me when this happens because I hate to lose someone especially when they are that close to stepping into some real freedom! You see she wanted me to carry her and like a responsible adult you cannot always carry the child. You must make them walk! The child will get mad at you because it knows you have the capability to carry them. But what they do not understand is that by you making them walk they will help develop their leg muscles so they will become strong. And soon not only will they be able to walk; they will be able to run! However I can only help those who are willing to help themselves but every time I lose one it hurts, that's just the way it is!

This brings us to Connie who has been my friend for over 30 years and Connie has the heart of a lioness! She is very brave, she has fear but she will not let that fear hold her back for long! She will always step up to the plate and do the right thing no matter how afraid she gets. She is an inspiration for me always and may god bless her! Not to long ago on the advice of a doctor Connie had an operation where the doctor removed a part of her feminine anatomy. After the operation she regretted having it done but she couldn't undo what was already done. So Connie made the best of it and went on with the business of living. Last year however she started having complications and this time the only recourse was an operation. The thought of this frighten her immensely. But like the lion heart she truly is Connie didn't go into doom and gloom thinking! Although she was frightened she kept her wits about her and went inside and contacted the Goddess within her. The wisdom she needed to make the right choices she prayed for and that Divine Mother answered her cry for help. She had the operation! I prayed for Connie and sent her healing every day before, during and after the operation. I did not want to lose one of my closest friends. I am a Psychic Medium so I have a little different view of death than most people; even so the thought of not having Connie or her husband "my little brother James" is just too painful for me to bear! The three of us received Knowledge from Maharaji " Prem Rawat" our first teacher together. And for 30 years we have been practicing meditation and are still going strong.

I was not the only person who prayed for Connie many of us did and I am happy to say that today she doing well. Whatever life throws her way she handles it with grace and dignity! It is a pleasure to know her and call her my friend! She has the heart of a lioness and has bravely faced death to overcome it and is still on her healing journey. She has courage and has truly stepped into womanhood! She is an example for all women wanting to take that same step!

As mentioned earlier I too was also a man who had not stepped into his manhood. Although I was grown up physically, mentally and emotionally I was still very immature. How did I allow this to happen? By living in my past and refusing to take responsibility for my life! My stepfather tried to kill me so please have pity on me! My mother didn't protect me so please give me sympathy! I have a right to blame them for messing up my life! It is not my fault it is all their responsibility-I am the victim here! By having this mindset although totally justified I was refusing to grow up and the only one I was hurting by doing this was me! This was the brutality of the truth I had to face to step into my manhood. Not only was I not loved by my parents, but one of them also tried to kill me! To step into manhood I had to let go of this and I had to forgive them both. This was painful because it was easier for me to be angry than it was to forgive them! Anger is a natural human emotion and we all get angry. There are many times when our anger is quite justified and I believed that my anger was totally justified. However it was too painful to deal with all of this anger so I repressed it. But just because I repressed it that did not mean that it had gone away! Once I began to do healing work on myself the anger came up to the surface. When it did I had to have the courage to take possession of it and own it; by doing so I was making myself whole again. I say this to you here because forgiveness was also a disowned part of me. As long as I held on to my position of not forgiving my parents I could not forgive myself! Part of my process of stepping into my adulthood was learning how to forgive my parents. And in doing so I was also coming to terms with learning how to forgiving myself. Also by doing so I was allowing myself to finally use my common sense to heal and grow!

If you are asking yourself at this point why this forgiveness stuff is so important, allow me to explain. I think you may see by now that I had very hostile emotions towards my stepfather however as a young boy there was not much I could do about my situation. I was not able to direct my anger towards him because he would have killed me, but the anger had to go somewhere. That anger redirected itself against me, yes you heard right against me! I blamed myself for being a coward and not standing up to my stepfather in spite of the fact that he was a grown man and I was but a young boy. I was not a coward just a young boy who could not understand why his father did not love him! When I finally came to terms with this anger I was able to forgive my stepfather for not loving me and trying to kill me. And also to embrace that young boy that was too afraid to stand up to that grown man who was hurting him! When I was able to let go then I began to heal and to make progress with my "Liver Cancer" because the input of toxic emotions I had been sending throughout my body and forcing my liver to process, were significantly reduced. As a result the overall condition of my health began to improve greatly!

This brings us to two other subjects also connected with forgiveness; the subject of self sabotage and the need to be perfect. It has been my experience that in the past whenever I committed self sabotage the two root causes were for me, guilt and the feeling of unworthiness. My feeling of unworthiness was tied in with the abuse inflicted upon me at a very early age as a child.

As already stated not being able to stand up to my abuser left me with the feeling of being a coward, and as a result of this I felt unworthy. In order to stop my self-sabotage I had to remove this belief! Forgiveness was the key to doing that! Time and time again I would set a goal and bust my back side to attain it and just as I was about to accomplish it, subconsciously I would do something to self destruct! Yet I would fail to see that it was all my own self- fulfilling prophesies! Until I was able to finally forgive that young boy for not being able to stand up to that adult who was hurting him; I was blind to this fact! However when I was finally able to let go of the past and forgive my parents and myself this behavior became crystal clear!

Forgiveness was of paramount importance in allowing me to see this fact! The need to be perfect was also rooted in the feeling of unworthiness due to abuse. No matter what I did nothing was ever good enough for my stepfather to embrace me with love! The harder I tried to win his approval the more I was rejected. In my young mind I believed that if I could only do things perfectly perhaps I would finally win his approval and love! However little did I realize no matter what I did this would never happened because this man hated me so much he tried to kill me! As I grew I began to become conscious of the fact that I was intelligent and my concept of what perfection is was coming from my mind, which is finite. A finite mind can never understand divine perfection but the heart can! When I was finally able to learn to forgive I realized that even in making mistakes the true perfection is recognizing those mistakes and then learning from them! You see if you can forgive yourself than you will be able to learn from your mistakes. If you do not allow forgiveness to manifest in your life then you cannot forgive others or yourself. As a result of that every time you make a mistake you might do what I did and inflict self punishment upon yourself with a vengeance! You see every time I made a mistake rather than learning and accepting the fact that mistakes are just part of the learning process, I would hear the voice of my stepfather in my head telling me how stupid I was for making the mistake! This would happen time and time again and I could even see myself doing this, but couldn't stop it until I finally found it in my heart to forgive! Then the need to be perfect also began to subside and so did the self punishment!

I might add here that if we had nothing to learn we would make no mistakes–but then what purpose would there be in us being on this earth? Although life may seem crazy at times everything is perfect and all is perfect rapture! Once I was able to let go of this need to be perfect I was open to allowing myself to be loved by myself and others. This not only brought more happiness into my life but also expedited my healing process. However this was the kind of work no doctor could do for me. I had to pay the price of facing my pain in order to heal from it! But if I was able to do this then it is not an impossible task and you can do it as well if you are willing to pay the price. Let me add here that I used a method developed by one of the teachers in the popular DVD the Secret; Hale Dwoskin it is called the Sedona Method™. I highly recommend it for releasing emotional issues past and present, as a matter of fact he calls this technique releasing because that's exactly what it allows you to do, release past and present traumas. If you would like to find out more simply go to www.sedonamethod.com ™.

I hope I have made it clear to you about the power of forgiveness in the healing process. Because if you can understand this you accelerate your healing process exponentially! Remember the old adage to err is human but to forgive is Divine! So let us forgive ourselves and get on with the business of living this life in totally abundant joy!

Chapter 17 – East Meets West

I decided to look back to see what I had learn thus far from my illness. One of the main factors was I now understood the power of the mind and its part in the trinity of the mind, body and emotions. The thoughts contained in my mind stream affect the content of my emotional body. These emotions have a direct affect on my physical body and how my body feels. Then there was the understanding of the emotional influences on my body and how important it is to feel good if you intend to heal yourself! Common sense tells you if are trying to assist your body back into health and harmony, the attitude you have within the content of your mind and the thoughts and emotions that they generate are of paramount importance to you! Awareness is the key to come from a position of power and clarity; understanding the fact that my personal will is an extremely powerful tool in the healing process as well. The will when used in tandem with the mind can manifest things on the physical plane of existence. And good health is one of those things it can manifest! The emotional journey along the way can be very enlightening. I had discovered the interplay between my thoughts and their affects on my body. I had learned how my thoughts were making me feel. I had transformed them to productive, healing and resourceful thoughts! And as result of doing so I now had the capability to focus on what I wanted to attract in my life, and then manifest it and you can as well! Then there was also coming into the understanding that my body is desperately doing everything in its power to keep me alive and healthy. And that my body and my breath are my two best friends.

Life has taught me through my illness many lessons that I could not have learned otherwise. How to listen and use my common sense to become a true friend to my body! And assist it any way I can in our healing process. I appreciate the breath that allows me to be able to maintain consciousness and life. This body is the home where my sprit resides, but it is running on a time factor! The more I expand in consciousness the more I appreciate this fact. The journey of self discovery is one of discovering my true nature. I am the son of a Mother who sustains me through the power of this breath of life! My Father's gift to me is the ever evolving consciousness that dares me to dream! It is through these dreams that we work our greatest magic. Dare to dream of the healthy body you desire. The breath of life vibrates within you therefore all miracles are possible! The restoration of my body back to good health begins with me and my mind. I must look at the reasons my choices, conscious or otherwise led me to a path of illness. This self analysis when done with honesty and compassion is healing to the soul and can open one up to the higher teachings. However none of any of this would be possible without the breath of life vibrating within me now. We must bring ourselves back into harmony with universal law! All true healing begins at this point. The gift of the body has been given. The gift of Consciousness has been given along with the gift of this Body. They are "Source Energy's" gift to me by which I am allowed to be in this earth school. They are a part of my greatest blessings!

I have learned that guidance can manifest in many ways. I must be watchful and open to the signs the universe may use to advise me.

Sometimes they can be quite obvious and sometimes they are not so obvious and lay hidden in the background. The key is that if a person is consciously looking for guidance the information that they need they will attract into their lives. It was now about six months since my last doctor's visit so I made an appointment to go in and be looked at. During the visit my doctor commented on how pleased she was with my improvement and spoke to about another interferon treatment. At that time it had been five years since my first treatment and she insisted that I was a perfect candidate for this new treatment. She said that improvements had been made and that rather than having to inject myself every other day, the newer treatment required only one injection a week, also the taking of some pills on a daily basis for the next six months. However she did honestly state that the treatment was still very painful! I told her I would have to think about it and that I would get back to her. I knew that my mind was already made up on this issue. I did not want to take the interferon treatment again! However I had prayed for guidance and I knew I just could not dismiss this without some reflection and introspection.

So I was going to ask my body what it wanted me to do. This may seem ridiculous to you. However if you are in touch with your body and have an open dialog with it, it does talk to you just not with words! So that night before I went to bed I took some quite time to relax and told my body I needed it to give me some assistance. Because I was not sure of what course of action to take on how I could help it heal. That night I had a dream that Bruce Lee and Chuck Norris were shaking hands at the coliseum in Rome. I knew exactly what this dream meant. The interpretation was a very simple one for me. You see for me in my mind Bruce Lee represented my Eastern healing techniques and Chuck Norris represented western medicine for me! They were not in conflict with one another, on the contrary they were shaking hands, and the East meets the West in harmony and friendship. I understood that my body had chosen to answer my question with a dream! Although I really did not want to, I knew I needed to take the interferon treatment once again because this was the guidance I was receiving from my body. This time the treatment along with myself-healing techniques would be enough to eradicate the virus, because this illness had nothing more left to teach me. I called the doctor the next morning and told her I was ready to start the treatment!

During the next six months of the interferon treatment I went from 200 lbs. to 150 lbs. I had no appetite what so ever; I actually had to force myself to eat. You see I was injecting a virus into my body which was the interferon, to kill another virus the Hepatitis-C! To say that this was taxing on my already debilitated body would be an understatement. I was very weak and could not walk very far without getting tired. The simplest things like shopping for food at the supermarket or doing laundry were very taxing on my body. My understanding of the mental body was of paramount importance to me in maintaining the proper mindset to promote the healing of my body at this time. I had to use the power of my mind and will to maintain the proper focus and mindset. I would only input myself with things that would keep me in the healing mindset.

By this time in my life I was alone again, the love of my life and I had separated. I mention this here because some of the things I began doing might have been cause for alarm for any person who might have been sharing my living space at the time. Let me explain what I mean. I began talking out loud to my body just like I would talk to another person who was in the room with me. I would ask my body questions like I was expecting it to answer, because I was! Now I know this may sound strange to most of you but I do not care if I sound strange! I had taken the road less traveled and I was setting the rules now; not my doctors or my friends or social protocol! I was going to use whatever worked for me and talking out loud to my best friend (my body) worked like a charm! I should also like to point out here that a dialog between my inner child and I had been taking place for a few years now. Needless to say there was a little emotional turmoil going on within me at this time! But I was not running away or trying to repress anything any longer, I was standing my ground and facing whatever came my way. However before I got better I got worse! That is just the way it worked out. It was during this time that I chose to look at my feeling about my own death! Death is not the subject of this book but to say that death never crossed my mind while I was going through all of this would be ridicules.

The native American Indians have a saying (*Hoca Hay*) it means today is a good day to die! Because for the native American Indians any day is a good day to be born, and any day is a good day to die! I have accepted this in my life and it has given me an immense sense of peace and freedom.

Never the less I knew I wanted to get on with my life and not my death! Talking to my inner child and my body was my way taking control of the situation. I needed to feel and believe that I was in control of my life and my health. That what I wanted was important–because to me it absolutely was. I was allowing myself to matter because I was bringing in a new mindset into the physical plane. You see I had been wrestling with this Hepatitis virus for twenty years and I had enough. Either it was going to kill me or I was going to kill it and I was not ready to die! I would not allow my body to be a host for this virus anymore. I had learned the lessons it had to teach me and now it was time for it to go! When I spoke to my body I often spoke to the virus as well, thanking it for being the catalyst for teaching me so many valuable lessons. I also was informing it that just like my time would come to die, it's time had come to die also!

I was laying my hands on myself and giving myself-healings every day, this help me feel like I was actively taking control of my own healing process. I was bringing in the Eastern modalities of esoteric healing and my doctor was bringing the Western science of modern medicine. Together we made up both barrels of a shotgun and the virus now didn't have a chance! About after the second month of the interferon treatment I began to feel a shift in the energy in my body. I knew it was a good shift because I felt a little better. I was not out of the woods yet but it was a step in the right direction and I knew it. Now my belief in myself and my healing process just got stronger. I was 100% convinced that there was nothing stopping my body and me from moving into perfect health! The affects of the interferon treatment became less painful as the months went by. By the sixth and final month I even started to get a little of my appetite back. This was a further indication to me that I was on the road to recovery. I was excited with the anticipation of living life in a healthy body! I was looking forward to doing many things that my illness prevented me from doing. I was looking forward to walking barefoot on the beach once again after twenty years–this would be my victory walk! Also to be able to have a great meal and enjoy a glass of wine, something I had not been able to do for years. These simple things most people take for granted that I had been denied for twenty years, I could now embrace and the gratitude I felt on many occasions brought me to tears!

The interferon treatment was now over and it was time for me to see my doctor again to get the results of the treatment. Blood tests were taken and about ten days later my doctor called me back in for the results. My doctor was smiling when I went into her office, this was a good sign I thought. As I had anticipated the virus was gone however my doctor told me not to get too happy just yet. After an interferon treatment the Hepatitis C Virus can return within the next six months! However if it does not return within those next six months, then it probably won't return at all she said. So I had to sit tight for six more months before I would finally know if my battle was finally over.

The following six months brought to light just how much of my life had been organized around my illness. Although I knew there was the possibility that the virus could return, I knew in my heart that it would not. I knew "Source Energy "did not help me get this far to allow me to relapse into sickness again! So I went on with my life as though the blessings of the miracle I had prayed for and that I was about to manifest, were going to stay with me for the rest of my life! I took the time to look back at the last twenty years of my life living with this Liver Cancer, to evaluate what I had truly learned by going through the process of healing from this disease. First and foremost my understanding of myself was enhanced! I knew who I was and what I was capable of accomplishing. My understanding of the relationship between me and my mind had grown stronger and clearer. And my ability to make my thoughts my allies as oppose to my enemies had also given me a sense of confidence in myself, that I had not known before in my life! Then there was the relationship between my mind and my emotions. I now knew with certainty that my thoughts affect my emotions, and that my emotions affect my body and my health. And I knew this experientially–not just mentally! Then there was the fact that I had become an accomplished healer who not only could help himself but also help others! I also had opened my psychic door and was also able to help people find closure over the loss of a loved one or a pet because I had become a medium. I saw my illness as a blessing that was the source for me to discover the gifts that Source-Energy had given to me! I also understood the power of gratitude! I cannot overstate the importance of gratitude in my life. The recognition of what is being given to us from that higher power and the appreciation of it, will allow us to attract more of what we want into our lives! Many people have died from Hepatitis C yet I was given a second chance and the gift of life, and for that I am truly grateful. Life is beautiful and I could have been given no greater gift than the gift of this life! Six months had passed, the time had come to see if the virus had made a comeback or not. I went to see the doctor for my results. As I walked into her office she had that smile on her face again. As she approached me and said only two words "it's gone"!

After getting the news from doctor I realized that my 20 year quest had come to an end. What I had set out to do I had successfully accomplished. Through the power of my will and intension I had beaten the odds! Through an in depth understanding of my mind; both conscious and subconscious and by the understanding of my inner child and emotional body, I overcame a premature death! By taking the road less traveled and following the inner guidance of my heart I have learned many priceless lessons. Sickness does not have to be a death sentence. It can be one of the most important teachers you will ever have in your life! With a simple shift of your focus you can see your illness as a blessing as opposed to damnation! You can see your body in a new light and redefine your relationship with your body temple! And by doing so the two of you can become best friends!

If I have gained nothing else from my experience of life on this earth, I have come to the earth plane and learned the lesson of love for myself and others. I hope my ancestors watching from the other side will appreciate my effort in learning this lesson. I hope my father the man I never knew and my stepfather the man who could never love me would be proud. I hope my Divine Father will finally allow me to come home into that heavenly abode and rest for a little while, until I must reincarnate again for my next set of lessons. I hope my Divine Mother is pleased with my effort and embraces me in love! For I do love her children and I have done my by best to elevate myself and the consciousness of my brothers and sisters on this planet!

I wish you good fortune and blessings on your healing journey.

Love Always.

James Arthur May

Source Reference Guide

Recommended Reading:
The Power of the Subconscious Mind by Joseph Murphy
The Law of Attraction by Esther and Jerry Hicks
Ask and It Is Given by Esther and Jerry Hicks You Can Heal
Your Life by Louise Hay
The Secret by Rhonda Byrne
The Spontaneous Healing Of Belief by Gregg Braden
The Astonishing Power of Emotions by Esther and Jerry
Hicks

Recommended Videos:
"The Secret"
"What the Bleep Do We Know?"

Recommended Audio:
The Holosync Solution™ www.centerpointe.com
The Sedona Method® www.sedonamethod.com
Teachings of Lazaris   www.lazaris.com

Recommended Meditation: ***Knowledge***!

www.wopg.org and www.findingout.org